The Truth About Building Muscle

Nutrition Book

By Jeffrey Bedeaux

The Truth About Building Muscle

Table of Contents

Detailed Table of Contents

Countless benefits to having good nutrition habits
The importance of drinking plenty of water
Having cheat days in your diet without guilt
Eating out
Power up your breakfast
During your sleep time
Alcohol and training
Beer data
Training + nutrition = mass, sample diet
Understanding food labels
1. Check the List of Ingredients
2. Pay Attention to Total Fat and Saturated Fat
3. Figure out the Percentage of Calories from Fat
Food label terms, what they really mean
10 biggest nutritional mistakes
1. Eating too much
2. Eating too little
3. Insufficient protein
4. Failing to cook for yourself
5. Not keeping a nutrition log
6. Too much fat & sugar
7. Not drinking enough water
8. Lacking positive nitrogen balance
9. Lacking food balance in meals
10. Ignoring supplementation
10 tips for eating well despite your busy schedule

Supplements

Protein shakes; these have to be your best friend
Total nutrition or complete meal replacement protein
Pure protein powder
Let's also talk about protein bars
Whey protein
Creatine: More than a sports nutrition supplement
What is creatine?
How does creatine work?
How to get the best gains from creatine
Creatine conclusion
Glutamine, the best amino acid

Vitamins and minerals

<u>Introduction</u>

About this book

Hello and welcome! Thanks for purchasing my new e-book. It's loaded with revolutionary proven knowledge and techniques that will allow you to quickly and efficiently transform your body to whatever level of fitness and muscularity you desire. You can do muscle toning or firming or conditioning for a sport or **even adding 20, 40, 60 pounds of new, hard muscle** to your frame. All without drugs and without spending a fortune on nutritional supplements and without wasting your time in the gym.

You see, a while ago my 25-year-old friend told me was getting into lifting weights at the gym and he wanted to know what I thought he should be doing in the gym to maximize his results. He knew that I wrote books on the subject, performed research on trainees from 16 to 82 years of age, measured the results every step of the way and synthesized them into full workouts and specialization workouts. He knew all that and more but he didn't want to read that much, he just wanted his best friend to tell him the core knowledge from all those books and all that research. The best of the best without any preamble, padding myself on the back or self-serving BS about how smart I was compared to others. So I gave it to him. Nothing more; nothing less.

That made me realize I really could condense what I've learned developing new data, feedback from customers, and experience from personal consultations. Everything into a book that I could make available to anyone in the world via the Internet.

And that's what you have right now. The best information garnered from years of research in real world testing. I urge you to read every word of it. The knowledge you need is in these pages and is laid out in a concise format and I don't repeat the same things over and over. That is with the exception of safety. Safety is the most important piece of information you can get out of this book. With that said I wouldn't dwell on it too much.

Getting the most from this book

If you are like most guys, you're tempted to turn to the chapters on workouts and dive right into your workouts with those killer techniques and principles. That's because most muscleheads see bodybuilding as merely hoisting weights up-and-down, over and over, slowly increasing the weight, under some misguided concept of this is what builds muscle. These are the guys who are always on the look out for the magic routine that has eluded them for so long. Don't make that mistake!

Now I know you're not going to like to hear this, but read this manual all the way through before beginning your program. I want you to get on the gym floor in the quickest time possible but I want you to be armed with the advanced knowledge needed to put that time to good use. If you skip a chapter thinking you already know everything needed to know about that training factor, you could be setting yourself up for a big disappointment. But don't worry I'll be there every step of the way.

We will be covering a lot of information in this book. Information that is anything but common knowledge even among the professional bodybuilders who rely on anabolic steroids for their massive gains. Well, there you have it. I've sufficiently warned you of the dangers of skipping ahead in this book and I've given you a couple of "extra emphasis" tools to make sure you get the most important details from all information I have jammed into these pages.

Also, you will notice a couple of inches of open space at the bottom of each page; I did this for a reason. I want you to write down and highlight the most important parts for you. This open space is for your notes. By reading and writing the ideas that really connect with you, you will be able to absorb and use those points without even being aware of it. Print out this book and write all over it; I want you to squeeze every benefit out of the huge amount of information within these pages.

Two other tools you will see throughout this book that will help you understand the key points are *The Doctor Says* dialog box and the *Doctor's Prescription* dialog box. Look for boxes like these as you are reading:

These 2 dialog boxes will help you get the most important information first. Also use them as a guideline for writing your own notes at the bottom of each page. After you have read this book you can skim through it later and read only the dialog boxes and your personal notes to re-connect with all the information contained in this book. I have found this technique to be very valuable to me when I want to skim a book I have already read and review the key points.

So here's what I want you to do now. If you have already been busting your ass in the gym training three to four days or more per week. Take a week off! You'll understand why later, but for now just plan on using that week to review this manual and fully prepare for your fiery return. If you're relatively new to bodybuilding, or it has been awhile since you've been in the gym, take the next week to introduce your body to what it's about to experience. In order to avoid overloading your body to the point of shutdown it's wise to begin a light exercise routine to prepare your muscles, joints and ligaments for the upcoming barrage. You don't want to go all out to the point you can barely move the next day. That would defeat the whole purpose of the first couple weeks of this program. Besides if you're looking for is an intense workout session, the real workout is coming up.

Dedication

This book is dedicated to every bodybuilder and athlete who has an acquiring rational mind; to every person who can throw off the chains of comfortable habit and unproven premises and move into new direction that is guided by reason and observational evidence, no matter where that direction takes him; to every person to try something immediately and thinks "How can I make this better?" To every person who is unafraid to challenge the false beliefs of the herd and lead others out of the cave and into the light.

In the world of bodybuilding it is these people with these genetics who are truly the greatest champions of the human race. To these people not just in the science of human strength but also in every science we all owe our enormous gratitude.

Why an e-book?

Some people ask me why I wrote this as an e-book. I could have written the draft of this book and taken to a mainstream book publisher, but there are a few reasons why I self published this as an e-book and they all benefit you.

Freedom of content: E-books can contain links to related material, special pages or even built-in programs. Also big publishing companies don't like controversy. They don't like writers being too blunt about certain topics. They prefer to re-edit or re-word certain things. With an e-book, which I both write and publish, I conclude whatever content I want to include. Which leads me to....

Freedom of style: Any writer does better when he uses his own "voice". For example, in a mainstream publication I would have to say, "many professional bodybuilders use dangerous drugs to augment their muscular development." But in my own e-book I can say, "pro bodybuilding is filled with unbridled use of every type of drug imaginable.

Steroids represent less than 10 percent of what drugs bodybuilders actually use today. The full truth is that they use up to 20 prescription drugs at the same time and 1000% of the recommended safe dose. They take drugs intended for diabetes, cancer, dwarfism, pain, bloating, cardiology, hematology, impotence; the list goes on and on.

Athletes and regular folks are dropping dead every year and the huge meltdown is coming because the real health effects (tumors, heart failure, kidney failure, etc) appear to take at least fifteen years to show up. Soon we'll be hearing about the failing health of the great names of bodybuilding from the '80s and '90s, if you haven't heard already." Try finding that kind of plain talk in a nice mainstream book. I'm sure you won't find it especially if the author puts down supplements anyway since that's where the real cash cow is in bodybuilding.

Freedom from templates: Mainstream publishers have a formula they have to follow. It is just the realities of the book business. Right now is the larger book format (9" x 11") with approximately 220 pages; it is all about shelf space in the bookstores and perceived value. So a new e-book with about 120 pages loaded with new ideas that's guaranteed to put 40 pounds of muscle on you doesn't have a prayer of getting into print, but a 220 page book showing women doing "workouts" with 3 pound dumbbells gets in every bookstore and featured every woman's magazine.

The perception of what is valuable is very different from what really has value in the gym. An e-book format allows me to get right to the point without adding a bunch of filler, such as lots and lots of pictures that you have already seen, to get the book up to 220 pages.

The amount of information packed into this e-book took 17 years to determine and compile. It can unlock the greatest muscle growth you've ever experienced. When

Einstein writes E=MC² on a piece of paper, it doesn't take a many pages but that knowledge can unlock enormous power.

Freedom of marketing: Digital content and the Internet is the wave of the future in publishing. When a mainstream book is published it gets an initial marketing push by the publisher and then it's all done. E-books can be promoted by links, banners, affiliate programs, and "word of mouse" that keep it in front of bodybuilders every day. Why should you care about that? The financial success of this e-book fuels the next one and that brings you more useful research information instead of the crap that's available in many books. As you can see in the bookstores, mainstream publishers say the same thing day after day, year after year.

Freedom of access: Less than 5% of the world's population lives in America. It can be pretty difficult and expensive to get an American book delivered to Turkey. But an e-book can be delivered around the world without extra costs and you can be reading it 20 seconds after you buy it.

And I'm not talking hypothetically here; this e-book not only sold copies in the United States and Canada, it also sold in the United Kingdom, France, Germany, Sweden, Switzerland, Australia, Brazil, Ireland, Singapore, South Africa, Denmark, Malaysia, China, Japan, Belarus, American Samoa and the Netherlands. All in the first 60 days!

Like the bodybuilders in the above countries around the world you're about to discover this e-book is absolutely loaded with useful information you can apply in your next workout. You're literally minutes away from the most productive workouts of your life.

Why I wrote this book

First let me explain why I wrote this book, I'll phrase it into a short story were I'm sure you can identify with the main character.

Let me introduce you to Average Joe. Joe is very typical of the bodybuilders trying to pack on muscle in today's gyms. Determined to look like "the huge guys" in the magazines, he signed up for his membership at the local gym, buys his weightlifting gloves and belt and all the other "essential tools" for packing on the pounds, and begins his quest.

At the gym he follows the lead of all the other "muscleheads" and begins bench pressing, curling, and squatting the most weight he can. Like the other misinformed Joes, he thinks that working harder and harder, steadily increasing the weight on the bar will force his body into growth beyond his wildest dreams. He makes some gains; enough to keep pushing on but soon finds himself stagnated.

Not seeing any more strength or size development Joe decides to go to the next level. He looks around the gym for the biggest iron pumping "consultant" he can find that also looks friendly enough to talk to. That guy is The Juice. Joe approaches Juice to inquire about the secrets to his bodybuilding. Juice tells Joe everything he knows about what exercises to choose, how much weight to use, what to eat and what "super supplements" to use.

Joe sets out again following everything Juice tells him; positive he now has the missing links to maximum growth. Some of what Juice told Joe was enough to move him out of his plateau temporarily. Within a few weeks he finds his strength and size stalemated again.

Frustrated Joe decides to turn to the "experts". He goes to the local bookstore and picks up every bodybuilding magazine they have and begins his research. Obviously with arms and legs the size of telephone poles and a chest the size of 2 Webster's dictionaries, anything these pros have to say must be gospel. Then there all the ads for the top-secret supplement discoveries promising you God-like powers from all the "latest" scientific research.

Confused and frustrated Joe spent a small fortune on supplements and is back in the gym. He is loaded with tips from all the pros and has so many "secret potions" running through his veins that he can be declared off-limits as a toxic waste dump! He makes a small gain, only to find it whither away as he hits "the wall". The wall is the place that all beginning and novice bodybuilders hit when they realize that building muscle is a whole lot harder than those hulking professionals in the magazines make it look.

Now comes the moment of truth. Here are the facts.

Fact: All those pro bodybuilders trying to coax you to purchase the next wave of natural supplements guaranteeing massive growth, got that big not from the natural supplements they are marketing but rather by pumping massive quantities of anabolic steroids into their veins.

Fact: The killer pre-contest and mass building routines those pros let you in on are enough to throw any bodybuilder into chronic overtraining without the aid of a serious dose of dangerous growth hormone and steroids. Or make you sick from a depressed immune system or seriously injure yourself.

Fact: The bodybuilding supplement market is a multi-multi-million dollar industry that is supported by well-intentioned serious seekers of muscle and fitness such as yourself, fall prey to the ads and articles designed for one thing, to take your hard earned money.

Fact: Supplement manufacturers and gym owners all follow the six-month rule of marketing. Basically six months is how long research has shown it takes the average "seeker of strength" to join a gym, purchase the supplements they're convinced they need, reach the wall where they see no more gains, get frustrated, and quit their workout program.

Fact: Those same bodybuilding magazines that projected air of "objectivity" actually own many of the supplements they're advertising and are recommending in their magazines.

Here are some of the worst offenders:

Flex Weider Supplements
Muscle & Fitness Weider Supplements
MuscleMag Muscle Tech
Muscular Development Twinlab
Muscle Media EAS

These companies weren't stupid. They realized early on that they could sell you a magazine full of great looking perfectly sculpted columns of muscle to make you feel puny and weak; then offer you ad after ad of expensive supplements with pumped up scientific claims to milk you for even more of your dough.

Be careful

Caution: This program involves a systemic progression of muscular overload that leads to lifting extremely heavy weights. As a result, a proper warm-up of muscles, tendons, ligaments, and joints is mandatory at beginning of every workout.

Warning: As this is a very intense program, it requires both a thorough knowledge of proper exercise form and a base level of strength fitness. Although exercise is very beneficial, the potential does exist for injury, especially if the trainee is not in good physical condition. As always consult with your physician before beginning any program of progressive weight training or exercise. If you feel any strain or pain when you start exercising, stop immediately and consult your physician.

<u>The building blocks</u>

I believe many of us make the process of bodybuilding far more complicated than it needs to be. This is especially true when it comes to nutrition. I've come to this conclusion after answering literally thousands of questions from bodybuilders for years. Through seminars, letters, phone consultations, and contact through the Internet, the same questions were asked and the same challenges were encountered over and over again. It didn't matter what level of experience, number of accomplishments, individual circumstances, or what part of the world a bodybuilder lived, when it comes to nutrition, our patterns of thinking and the obstacles they faced were basically the same.

As I strive to strengthen my skills as an effective bodybuilding coach, one of my goals is to simplify the bodybuilding process. The bottom line is that **we are all after the same things; to build muscle, lose body fat, or a combination** of building muscle and losing body fat. We also want to do so in the most efficient ways and in the shortest period of time.

If you embrace the nutritional strategies I've outlined in this book, how you need to build muscle and lose body fat will be simpler. **Notice the word I used was *simple*—not easy!** Nothing is easy; nothing worth having, anyway. Eating to create a lean and muscular physique is no exception.

Why you need good nutrition

If you want to produce high-quality muscle and maintain lower body fat levels from the time and effort you invest in training, you *must* feed yourself properly. Many experts feel the way you eat accounts for as much as 50 percent of the way you look. If you want an impressive muscular body, you are going to have to pay close attention to what you are eating.

Sound nutrition is that important to your bodybuilding efforts. A heavy emphasis needs to be placed on studying winning nutritional strategies and executing those strategies on a consistent basis.

Motivation builds the foundation of good eating habits

"I'm so confused about nutrition!" many bodybuilders often complain. "My training is great but, when it comes to how I should eat, I don't have a clue!"

Good eating habits are built upon a foundation of motivation. Let's get honest with ourselves for a moment. Is the difficulty in this particular situation in *understanding* nutrition? Or, is the real challenge *following through* with eating the way we already know we should?

Let's admit what's really going on in some of our minds. Eating delicious foods is one of life's simplest, easiest-to-attain, and greatest pleasures. Sometimes, it's very difficult to stay away from food that doesn't support our bodybuilding efforts. Great-tasting and unhealthy food becomes too much of a temptation for us. Even when we are committed to eating properly, it's sometimes too difficult to break away from our busy schedules and eat our meals at all; whether they are good for us or not.

Doctor's Prescription:
Keep your nutrition sound and your other physique goals will come to you much easier.

The key to eating to build muscle comes down to being properly motivated to do so. Because you are taking the time to read this nutritional advice, I assume you're pretty motivated. This is a great time to determine exactly why *today* is the day you'll make the commitment to earn the physique you really want by eating right. If you know *why* you want to do something, figuring out *how* to do it will become much easier. You must first take care of figuring out *why* and, hopefully, my advice will help you figure out *how* to meet your physique enhancing goals.

Eating to build muscle and lose body fat is a *way of thinking* just as much as it is a series of actions. Many bodybuilders get easily confused, frustrated, and eventually overwhelmed with the subject of proper nutrition. Rock-solid bodybuilding nutrition doesn't need to be complicated in order to be effective.

Three important keys to understanding effective nutrition

Let's break down and simplify this important aspect of bodybuilding. You basically need to understand three things about nutrition:

1. The main purpose for each of the three macronutrients: Protein, carbohydrates, and fat

2. The "right" ratio, or the "correct" percentages, of protein, carbohydrates, and fat that your food should be divided into in order to meet your bodybuilding goals

3. The number of calories you should consume to meet your specific physique-enhancement goals

Good nutrition seems much easier when it is broken down and you look it at from that perspective, doesn't it? But what do the three macronutrients do for our bodies? What ratio of our food should be allocated to protein, carbohydrates, and fat? How do I determine how many calories I should eat? I'll answer those questions—and a whole lot more.

Those questions about nutrition provide a wide range of answers that are not necessarily easy to find. Unfortunately, there are no easier ways around this fact. There are no magic numbers, solutions, or formulas that I, nor anyone else, can give you to make the process effortless; no matter what you are told. These answers not only vary from person to person, they also can vary within the very same *person* during different periods of time.

With simplicity and efficiency in mind, let's discuss the macronutrients. In general terms, all food is broken down into three major groups of macronutrients; protein, carbohydrates, and fat. Here is a simple explanation of what they are and what each of them does for our bodies:

Protein, your #1 priority

Protein, far and away, is the most important nutrient you'll need to build muscle on your body. **Muscle *is* protein. Protein *is* muscle.** Without enough protein, you'll have a very difficult time seeing results from your training. Plain and simple, you're simply not going to grow muscle without a sufficient amount of protein.

It is important for you to maintain a balance in the positive flow of nitrogen on a consistent basis. By this, I mean you absolutely *must* consume more nitrogen than you excrete. You need to keep your body in a positive protein accrual environment. If you happen to be excreting more nitrogen than you consume, it doesn't matter. I have discovered, like many other bodybuilders, the more protein I consume the bigger and stronger I get.

How much protein should I eat to build muscle?

How much is the "right" amount of protein to eat each day, you ask? 100 grams? 250 grams? 500 grams? You will need to *experiment* to determine what the proper amount of protein is that will keep you in a positive protein accrual environment.

Bodybuilders should start with a gram per pound of bodyweight—and move *upwards* from there. Many experts estimate this is how much the average hard-training bodybuilder needs per day. My only suggestion would be, if your body can efficiently use more, then by all means, give it more and build more muscle!

The Doctor Says:
Protein is the most important piece of your nutrition program. Always have some protein in each meal so you will have a constant flow of amino acids in your system. This alone will help you keep your hard earned muscle while at the same time you can add on more mass.

There is also a very old, outdated, and conservative method of determining the "proper" amount of protein you should ingest. Unfortunately, too many bodybuilders hold on tightly to this theory. I don't believe there is any way possible this cookie cutter rule can apply to everyone; especially every single hard-training bodybuilder. This method suggests that you multiply your body weight in kilograms times 1.5 to figure the grams of protein to consume daily. FYI - divide your weight in pounds by 2.2 to determine how much you weigh in kilograms.

The only reason I even include this guideline is because 9 out of 10 people in the bodybuilding world are going to tell you this is the "right" amount of protein; not a single gram more! If you ingest any more protein than that, they warn, you are going to damage your kidneys.

I suggest you shouldn't be so conservative about your protein consumption; especially if you want to make the most use of your hard training and pack on some serious, rock-solid muscle mass! But, if you do try this widely accepted formula, be sure to experiment upwards from there. If you are able to handle more than that amount efficiently, you will probably gain more muscle. One thing you don't want to do is rob yourself of even one more ounce of precious muscle!

"How much protein should I eat then? I calculate my total should be 177 grams a day." Bodybuilder A says. I recommend determining the amount of protein you should eat a little differently. Instead of figuring out the total grams of protein you can efficiently digest in the entire day; **determine how much you can efficiently digest at each meal.**

Why? If you eat your daily total, let's say, of 300 grams of protein in *four* meals as opposed to 7, the efficiency of how your body digests that protein would differ, wouldn't it?

If you take those 300 grams of protein and divide that total by four meals, that would equal 75 grams per meal. Those 300 grams of protein divided by 7 meals equals 43 grams per meal. Obviously, your body will have a much easier time digesting the 43 grams per meal than it would 75 grams. You are eating the very same amount of protein for the entire day—but are creating a big difference in the efficiency of its digestion and utilization. **Your body would have a much easier time using the protein to help build muscle if it was spaced out evenly throughout the day.**

Let me ask you a question: Are you confused about the amount of protein some experts in the bodybuilding community are recommending? You really should be more concerned with consistently eating more frequent, high-protein meals and properly spacing them throughout your day. The average meal replacement contains about 40 grams of protein. Even those people who don't think the human body can assimilate large amounts of protein will agree that it can digest 40 grams every two to three hours, right?

Every two to three hours creates what I call a **"Protein Window of Opportunity."** The more of these opportunities you take advantage of; the more you will augment your efforts in the gym. The more you consume high-quality protein during these windows— regardless of the amount of protein in that "window" or daily total of protein you think your body needs—the more muscle you will build. The key to successfully building muscle is eating smaller, more frequent meals throughout the day. Instead of worrying about that often-debated daily total of protein, break it down into two-hour to three-hour increments.

Doctor's Prescription:
Space out your protein consumption throughout the day to allow your body to assimilate as much protein as possible. This way you won't be sending your protein (and hard earned cash) right down the toilet.

Do the math. The guy who eats 7 meals as opposed to four meals a day has almost twice as many "Protein Windows of Opportunity" to take advantage of. Four a day, times seven days a week, equals 21 more "windows." Every month that's 91 more and every year the total grows to an incredible 1,092 more "Protein Windows of Opportunity" that are used. All other factors being the same, who do you think will build more muscle over the course of that year?

Good protein sources

Food	Serving Size	Calories	Protein (g)	% cal. from protein
Whey protein	1 scoop	100	24	96
Egg whites	6	102	24	95
Turkey breast	6 oz.	180	40	89
Tuna	6 oz.	180	39	87
Ground turkey	6 oz.	220	48	87
Chicken breast	6 oz.	180	36	80
Sirloin steak	6 oz.	345	51	59
Chicken thigh	6 oz.	330	36	51
Lean ground beef	6 oz.	435	45	43
Pork	6 oz.	315	24	31
Ground beef	6 oz.	270	15	23
Salmon	6 oz.	300	42	56
Eggs	1	75	6	34
Peanuts	1 oz.	90	4	18
Yogurt	8 oz.	120	13	43
Skim milk	8 oz.	90	9	40
Swiss cheese	1 oz.	90	8	35
2% milk	8 oz.	120	8	27
cheddar cheese	1 oz.	110	7	25
Whole milk	8 oz.	150	8	21

The danger of eating too much protein

Is eating too much protein dangerous? Many experts will tell you that eating too much protein will cause damage to your kidneys. Obviously, by the amount of protein I've been eating consistently every single day throughout my life, I either don't believe this is true or I am willing to take the risk in order to reach my ambitious bodybuilding goals. Besides, according to medical journals, you would have to eat 600+ grams of protein per day for a long time to have an effect on your kidneys.

Do I think, regardless of what the experts say you should ingest a large amount of protein like I choose to do? I can't make that decision for you. I can, however, share with you the reason why I do despite some people's warnings. The people that I trust to give me accurate information tell me there are no scientific studies to back up those doom-and-gloom claims. They have theorized that the experts have come to their conclusion because the kidneys play a major role in the synthesizing of protein. Thus, if they are forced to do more work than the average person, they are at a greater risk to suffer damage.

I, myself, haven't had any problems. I always make sure I do the things doctors recommend to help your body digest the protein like drinking a lot of water.

I am certain, however, that I have built a significant amount of muscle mass every single year that I've been training. I attribute much of that to **consistently eating high-quality protein** day after day, week after week, month after month, and year after year.

I firmly believe my body is able to assimilate most of the 300 grams I eat every day. There are studies that suggest the **hard training athletes can efficiently assimilate up to a whopping 72 grams of protein at a time.** That's far more than the old "multiply your body weight in kilograms times 1.5" formula!

I choose to take my chances, but you should talk to your physician if you have any concerns about eating excessive amounts of protein. I don't know anything about the effects of "excess" protein for certain. You'll need to make the decision of exactly how much protein to eat for yourself.

Carbohydrates, the energy you need

Carbohydrates give you the energy to train hard in the gym and carry out your everyday activities. Your body needs carbohydrates on a consistent basis throughout the day to feed the brain, which uses glucose, or blood sugar, as its primary energy source. Glucose is a carbohydrate used by every cell in the body as fuel.

When carbohydrates stored in the body are depleted too far, the body will convert precious muscle-building protein into glucose instead of regular carbohydrates to give the body the energy it needs. As a bodybuilder, you want to do everything you possibly can to avoid this from occurring. The very last thing you want is to have your hard-earned muscle mass sacrificed for energy. Consuming enough carbohydrates will prevent this from happening.

Excess carbohydrates, however, will be converted into fat. How can you avoid eating too many carbohydrates? I was once offered a suggestion I found to be very helpful. The strategy was to **eat the majority of carbohydrates in the morning and immediately after working out.** These are ideal times for the body to process carbohydrates more rapidly.

Some people believe you should limit your carbohydrate consumption after 6 or 7 p.m. They believe carbohydrates are converted to body fat much easier at that time because of your body's ability to burn fat is reduced while sleeping. Others have a different opinion. They believe it doesn't matter when you eat your carbohydrates. The body processes carbohydrates the same all the time.

The Doctor Says:
You will need to experiment with your carb consumption. Everybody is different so there isn't a cookie cutter program that will work for everyone. It goes without

saying but, experiment with the healthy carbohydrates; we all know what a candy bar will do (or not do) for your training.

Personally, I agree with the latter opinion. Carbohydrates in the morning, carbohydrates in the evening, or carbohydrates in the afternoon, in my opinion, it ultimately doesn't matter when you eat them. What is important is, at the end of the day, the calories that you've burned are greater than the calories you've consumed.

How do you determine the "right" amount of carbohydrates you should eat? I decide the amount of carbohydrates I'll eat this way:

As a bodybuilder, I will *always* keep my protein intake high to build muscle (usually, this is about 300 grams a day). If I'm trying to get lean or stay lean, I will closely monitor the fat in my diet. I also realize I must stay within a certain calorie range to meet my personal goals. What's left to consider? Only carbohydrates. I eat enough carbohydrates to give me just enough energy to train heavy and with intensity, have enough energy to do my regular life's activities, and to manage my body fat level. After I total the calories from my essential protein and incidental fat, the calories coming from carbohydrates can't cause me to exceed the total calories I've allotted myself for the day. The calories derived from carbohydrates must "sandwich" in between.

Starchy carbohydrates, stay away from them

As I work with more bodybuilders from around the world, I'm beginning to realize the biggest problem for most of us is over eating starchy or grainy carbohydrates. I think the biggest problem with starchy, complex carbohydrates is that they are very easy to overeat. It doesn't take very much rice or pasta to add up to a lot of calories.

You don't get very much food in a single serving of starchy carbohydrates; especially for the amount of calories that one serving contains. One serving of white rice contains about 150 calories and about 35 grams of carbohydrates. One serving of rice adds up to a puny 3/4 of a cup—and that's after it's cooked! That's not very much food.

How often do you stop after eating only 3/4 of a cup of cooked white rice when you are hungry, really? "Whoops, I guess I put a little too much in that measuring cup. Oh well." I know how it goes; I've been there too! I think the reason why a lot of bodybuilders who eat "clean" but can't get lean as quickly as they want or even stay fat is because they're unaware of overeating starchy carbohydrates.

I tend to lose body fat more quickly when I avoid starchy carbohydrates altogether. I believe the reason why is because I ingest fewer *calories* by replacing them with vegetables, or fibrous carbohydrates. You can eat an entire 16-ounce bag of broccoli has only 175 calories and 20 grams of carbohydrates.

I used to believe avoiding carbohydrates like rice, potatoes, oatmeal, and pasta and substituting them for vegetables was better for fat loss because I thought different types carbohydrates were digested a lot differently. I now feel that it's all a matter of calories burned versus calories ingested. That's how you effectively lose body fat. It doesn't matter which kind of carbohydrates you eat.

You should get your hands on a calorie-conversion book and look up just exactly what is considered a serving of your favorite carbohydrate, and more importantly, exactly how many calories that serving contains. In many cases, you'll be surprised just how small the serving is and how large the number of calories it contains. When dieting strictly, what type of foods do you crave the most and find the most satisfying? If you are like me, it's definitely complex carbohydrates!

Choose the right carbs at the right time

Slow-digesting carbs: You will want to use slow-digesting carbs for a large portion of your carb intake since they give you a slow and steady supply of energy. They also maintain a steady release of insulin which aids in the control of bodyfat levels.

Good selections of slow-digesting carbs:

- Apples
- Beans
- Brown rice
- Cream of rye cereal
- Oatmeal
- Oat bran cereal
- Oranges
- Red potatoes
- Rye bread
- Seven-grain bread
- Yogurt

Medium-digesting carbs: You should also make medium-digesting carbs a big part of your diet. They are called the "in-between-carbs" since they neither shoot into the bloodstream nor trickle in the way slow-digesting carbs do. Starchy carbs, which make up most of the calories eaten by people, also fall into this category.

Good selections of medium-digesting carbs:

- Buckwheat pancakes
- Corn
- Most fruit
- Honey
- Peas

White rice

Most pasta

Yams

Fast-digesting-carbs: Sugar and other simple carbs fit into this category because they hit the bloodstream rapidly. They are most helpful after training when your muscles are starving for nutrients and need energy ASAP. Throughout the rest of the day it is a good idea to keep your consumption of fast-digesting carbs to a minimum.

Good selections of fast-digesting carbs:

Cold cereals

Cream of rice

Cream of wheat

Gatorade

Potatoes

Pop

White bread

Bagels

Here I'll break down the carb information a little more: These charts will separate carbs by complex, fruit, and vegetable types.

Complex carbs chart

Food	Serving	Carbs (g)
Black beans	3 oz dry	20
Brown rice	1.5 oz dry	20
Multigrain bread	1 slice	20
Oatmeal	3 oz dry	20
Pasta	1 oz dry	20
Pinto beans	2 oz dry	20
Potatoes	4 oz baked	20
White rice	1 oz dry	20

Fruit chart

Food	Serving	Carbs (g)
Apple	1 medium	20
Banana	1 medium	20
Cherries	1 cup	20
Orange	1 medium	20
Peaches	2 medium	20
Pear	1 medium	20
Pineapple	5 oz	20
Watermelon	10 oz	20

Vegetable chart

Food	Serving	Carbs (g)
Broccoli	1 cup	10
Carrots	5 oz	10
Cauliflower	2 cups	10
Green peppers	2 medium	10
Peas	0.5 cup	10
Spinach	1 cup	10
Yellow squash	1 cup	10

Fats, they aren't all bad

Fat in your diet serves a vital purpose for the body. Fat acts as a structural component for all cell membranes and supplies necessary chemical substrates for hormonal production. Fat protects vital organs and carries fat-soluble vitamins. **Your body needs fat so don't try to avoid it completely.** Many experts feel that 10-20 percent of your total dietary calories should come from fat.

Why does every package of cottage cheese, milk, dressing, or yogurt make this huge deal of it's low fat content, usually deceptively advertised as: "98% fat free!" which still could mean that a considerable chunk of the calories from the product comes from fat. Who cares? The words: "Fat Free" sells like crazy.

The reason for this is obvious - we have been in a state of complete media overload, hammered with messages about how bad fats are for us, on a daily basis for many years now. Bodyfat, cardiovascular disease, diabetes... You know the list.

Fat isn't the devil. In fact, you'd get sick, malnourished, and eventually die if it wasn't for the fat in your food. You need it, period. Like with everything else, it's only a matter of keeping things in a proper perspective, and maintain a healthy balance.

One thing that is true about fat is that it is the biggest bandit around when it comes to packing calories. **For every gram of fat you eat, you get more than twice as many calories as a gram of protein or carbs.** Fats have 9 calories per gram as opposed to 4 calories per gram for the others.

You have to look at the big picture when you review your fat intake. What does it consist of? Saturated, unsaturated, or polyunsaturated fat? If there's plenty of the first, and little of the two latter, it's time for you to consider your eating habits. As a rule of thumb, it's the saturated fat that causes most of the trouble for people. Granted - all three categories yield the same number of calories - but they are very different when it comes to what they do once inside your body.

Saturated fats are found in animal sources, such as meat, egg yolks, milk, and peanuts and coconuts. These are the nasty little creeps that clog up your arteries, most readily settle in on your midsection, and generally do their best to mess your health up.

The "good" fats, on the other hand, are found mostly in vegetables and fish. **Olive oil, flax seed oil, and fish oil are prime examples of good sources for "good" fat.** However, make note that we're talking fish oil, not fish **liver** oil here. Fish liver oil may contain massive doses of vitamin A, which is fat-soluble and can be toxic if overdosed. Not cyanide, drop-dead toxic, but the kind of thing that could make you pretty sick and miserable if consistently overdosed over a period of time.

So what are the benefits of fat? For one, we have the essential fatty acids (EFA). As the name implies, these are essential for your survival, just like any vitamin or mineral. In short, they're part of the big puzzle that keeps you alive an' kicking, pal! **Fish oils are generally very good sources of EFAs.**

Secondly, fat is needed to absorb the fat-soluble vitamins from the food you eat. Without the fat, the vitamins go out the natural way. Without fat, absorbing fat-soluble vitamins is like trying to fetch water without a bucket. Last but not least, fat is what adds most of the flavor to your food. Without fat, most of what you eat would be pretty bland and boring.

Fat is good for you, as long as you don't take it overboard. Any less and you're most likely not getting enough. Any more, and you run the risk of packing on the love handles. And of the fat you DO eat, always strive to keep as much of it to be from the poly- and unsaturated fats. Don't go nuts about having a yolk or some peanut-butter once in a while, it's perfectly Ok as long as you don't lose sight of the big picture.

Reducing fat in your diet

By now you know that too much fat—especially saturated fat—is not good for you. Your body can easily store excess calories from fat as body fat. Plus, saturated fats from animal products, such as meats and dairy foods, can clog your arteries and contribute to heart disease.

But be careful. Although reducing dietary fat is important, eliminating all fat from your diet is not at all healthy. Fat is an essential nutrient that produces energy for daily activities and supplies the body with vitamins A, D and E, which are needed for healthy skin and optimal growth. The body cannot produce fat on its own; it must be provided through dietary intake. For these reasons you should enjoy some fats in your diet, especially monounsaturated fats like olive oil. The key is moderation—not elimination.

Research indicates that an excessive intake of saturated fats tends to raise blood cholesterol levels, thereby increasing risk for heart disease. Animal products—such as beef, butter, dairy products and lard—typically contain more saturated fat than do vegetable products. But some vegetable oils, such as coconut and palm oil (also known as tropical oils), contain large amounts of saturated fat.

There's also an unclassified newcomer in the fat realm—trans fatty acid. Trans fatty acids are the end products of a process called hydrogenation, in which vegetable oils are hardened. The implications that trans fatty acids may play a negative role on health is currently being reviewed, but many nutrition professionals are already advising a limited intake.

Health authorities recommend that Americans consume 20 percent or less of their total daily calories from fat, with 10 percent or less of those calories from saturated fat. Use the Nutrition Facts panel on food labels to help determine how much fat is in food. The following chart can help guide your fat intake. Determine how many calories are in your diet and use the chart to discover how many grams of fat are in 20 percent and 10 percent of your calorie intake. Remember, the recommended percentages refer to your total fat intake over time, not the fat in single foods or meals.

Calories per Day	Total Fat per Day (grams)	Total Saturated Fat per Day (grams)
1,200	26 or less	13 or less
1,600	36 or less	18 or less
2,000	44 or less	22 or less
2,200	48 or less	24 or less
2,500	54 or less	27 or less

10 tips to reduce fat

To help cut down on your fat intake, use the following tips when preparing foods:

1. Use evaporated skim milk instead of cream when preparing sauces or desserts.

2. Create your own nonfat salad dressing by mixing balsamic vinegar, mustard and herbs. If you really prefer an oil-based dressing, try using three parts vinegar to one part oil.

3. Drain nonfat yogurt through a sieve or cheesecloth overnight in the refrigerator, and use in recipes that call for cream.

4. Saute foods in chicken broth, vegetable stock, tomato juice or wine instead of frying them in oil or butter.

5. Keep olive oil in a spray bottle to a lightly coat sautÉ pans.

6. You can make your own taco shells. Hang soft corn tortillas directly over the oven rack (with the sides of the tortilla hanging down) and bake at 400 degrees until they're crisp. (Taco shells sold in supermarkets are usually fried.)

7. Whip up your own french fries. Place 1/4-inch-thick potato slices on a nonstick baking pan and coat with a light spray of oil. Sprinkle with paprika or salt, and bake at 350 degrees for 35 to 40 minutes. Turn once during baking.

8. To maximize flavor, toast nuts before baking with them. That way, you'll be able to use less. Or sprinkle nuts on top of a home-baked dessert instead of mixing them into the batter.

9. Substitute six egg whites plus one whole egg for every three eggs in your favorite recipes.

10. Substitute an equal amount of applesauce or any baby-food fruits for up to half of the total oil in your favorite dessert recipes. Strained prunes actually enhance the chocolate flavor in brownies!

Why eating excess fat makes us fat

While most of us know that consuming excessive amounts of fat will make us fat, we don't all understand exactly why this is true. To implement a successful weight management program, you need a good understanding of fat and why this nutrient makes us fat.

The amount of energy a particular food has depends on the quantity of fat, carbohydrates, and protein it contains. Food energy, both in its consumption and expenditure, is measured in terms of calories. Foods are either made up of fats, protein, carbohydrates, or a combination. A food that contains mostly fat will contain more than twice the calories than a food containing mostly carbohydrates and/or protein. For example, compare a serving of low-fat yogurt to a serving of nonfat yogurt—the low-fat yogurt has quite a few more calories than the nonfat variety because every gram of fat has more than twice the calories of a gram of protein or carbohydrate.

No more than 20 percent of your total calories should come from fat, fewer than 10 percent from saturated fat, the most damaging form. A recent study of 23 lean men and 23 obese men found little difference in the total number of calories each group consumed. But the obese men consumed, on average, more than 33 percent of their total calories from fat, compared with 19 percent for the lean men. Because the body converts dietary fat into body fat more easily than it converts protein and carbohydrates into body fat, the obese men were storing more fat even though both groups consumed the same total number of calories.

During the process of converting protein and carbohydrates to fat, your body uses them as energy and burns more than a quarter of their calories; it takes more energy (calories "burned") to convert carbohydrates and protein into body fat than it does to convert dietary fat into body fat. Thus, more carbohydrate and protein calories are used and fewer are stored as fat. Dietary fat, on the other hand, goes straight into storage, with very few calories being used. For example, Joe consumes 2,000 calories a day of which 40 percent come from fat. If Joe replaces half of the fat calories (20 percent of total calories) with calories coming from complex carbohydrates, less food will be converted to body fat even though the total number of calories consumed has not changed.

It is important to note that when that 20 percent of the 2,000 calories from fat now comes from carbohydrates (or protein), you consume a lot more food, since each gram of carbohydrate or protein contains less than half as many calories per gram. Therefore, when you begin to decrease the amount of fat in your diet and replace it with carbohydrates and protein, even if you still consume the same amount of food as before, you will be consuming a lot fewer calories.

If dietary fat were easy to control, most "diets" would probably succeed. Even with the recent explosion of low-fat and nonfat products, people generally still eat too much fat. The reason is simple: We have grown up loving fat, and we are accustomed to its taste and texture. Although most people do not usually crave fat as they do sugar or salty foods, we do have a strong taste preference for fat. Fat is responsible for the flavor and texture of many of our favorite foods: meats, cheese, dressings, sauces, creams, desserts, etc.

Because a high-fat diet increases fat storage and yields more than twice the amount of calories, the most effective way to reduce body fat is to concentrate on reducing your daily fat intake. Even if you do not consciously lower your total caloric intake, making the switch to a low-fat diet will most likely result in fat loss. However, attempts to suddenly restrict high-fat foods when you still have a strong preference for them causes feelings of deprivation which may, in turn, cause a higher intake of fat than normal. Deprivation is part of the "diet" process, and one of the main reasons it is doomed to fail. It is very important to make gradual, healthier changes to the foods you enjoy.

Drastic changes backfire. When people base their food choices on the number of calories consumed and a "foods allowed/not allowed" list, the focus is on numbers rather than satiety and enjoyment of the foods' taste and texture. This often negates any positive effect the original focus on choosing low-fat foods may have had. Simply counting calories and grams of fat does not make for a permanent healthy lifestyle change. If tastes do not shift to enjoying foods lower in fat, this quickly becomes too restrictive and normal eating habits resume.

I'm not saying that you should avoid counting grams of fat altogether. The way to lower fat in your diet is to become a fat-conscious eater—and this requires that you know the amount of fat in each food. However, instead of counting fat grams and deciding if it is a "good food" or a "bad food," try to balance the foods you are eating so that you average 20 percent or less of your total calories from fat each day. It's okay to have a piece or two of high-fat pizza if you are truly hungry and craving it, as long as you balance that out with low-fat foods at other meals soon after. What's crucial is to learn how to make small healthier changes. Consume fat in moderation by balancing higher fat foods with lower fat foods.

You should now have a better understanding of fat and why excess consumption of this nutrient makes us fat. Your greatest challenge, however, is not learning new low-fat shopping or cooking techniques. Nor is it remembering how to calculate fat percentages or what to say to the waiter to reduce the fat in your restaurant meal. The greatest challenge facing you at this moment is deciding whether you are willing to make a change—to make small, gradual changes to the foods you love.

Sure, there is plenty of work to be done, but it really doesn't matter how long this new process takes. If you allow changes to take place over several years, your body will adjust comfortably, and you will be more likely to maintain the healthy lifestyle permanently. When you begin achieving improvements in energy and physical and psychological performance, the fun and excitement you experience will make the change well worth the effort. Action creates motivation!

What is the best ratio of macronutrtients?

Let start off by saying there is no "right" answer. The experts in the health and fitness community often debate the recommended ratio, of protein, carbohydrates, and fat to effectively build muscle and lose body fat. The amount you need is based on your own body's ability to metabolize nutrients and on your particular fitness goals. Again, experimentation is needed on your part here.

Don't get overwhelmed by trying to nail down an exact percentage! In the big picture, over the course of time a 10 percent difference or swing in a couple of the macronutrients is really not a big deal; especially if it causes you to procrastinate from starting your diet! If you are truly committed, you will have plenty of time to make adjustments when you pay close attention to your body.

This is how I keep it simple in my mind: As a bodybuilder, I must eat more protein than an average person. My secondary focus is consuming enough carbohydrates to have enough energy to train hard, prevent the body from ever using muscle as an energy source, and fuel my regular lifestyle activities. I sometimes add fat to my diet for energy or eliminate it altogether depending on how lean I want to be at the time.

From that basic rationale, you can see that I don't necessarily worry about an exact ratio of macronutrients to gain quality muscle mass and reduce body fat. **The percentages, however, normally end up being around 50 percent protein, 35 percent carbohydrates, and 15 percent fat.**

Meals; how many per day should I eat?

After you've estimated the total amount of calories that you need to eat each day, decided on the right ratio of protein, carbohydrates, and fat, you need to commit to an eating schedule, which spreads that food evenly throughout the day.

How many meals should you eat? That will depend on your time constraints and the total daily calories you allow yourself to eat. **A good rule of thumb would be to eat smaller, more frequent meals.** A dedicated bodybuilder should eat *at least* five times a day and space those meals no further than three hours apart.

Doctor's Prescription:

Depending on your schedule, make sure you eat 5-7 meals per day. Spread out your protein consumption evenly over the meals so you can keep a constant flow of amino acids in your system.

I eat 7 meals a day that are spread out every 2.5 hours. I've been eating this way for years. It's difficult at times because eating so frequently interrupts my train of thought and activities. But, because I am committed to becoming the best drug-free bodybuilder that I can be, that's a price I'm willing to pay.

The theory behind this way of eating is this: I have found eating smaller, more frequent meals, or in other words **"grazing" throughout the day, is the most efficient way for my body to process food.** Even though I may eat 7 meals a day, my total amount of calories of those meals only adds up to around 2,700 - 3,200 calories. 7 meals, totaling 3,000 calories, are far more efficient for the body to handle than only three meals totaling 3,000 calories.

Calculate the amount of protein, carbs, and fat in food

Before calculating the percentages of each of the macronutrients (protein, carbohydrates, and fat) make up of your total food intake, you must know the calorie conversion of each of them. A calorie is a unit to state the heat content of food. In simple terms, it is the amount of energy needed to "burn up" that type of food and amount of food.

Calorie Conversion

One calorie of protein is equal to 4 grams.
One calorie of carbohydrate is equal to 4 grams.
One calorie of fat is equal to 9 grams.

If you want 50 percent of the 2,500 calories you've allowed yourself for the day to come from protein, simply multiply 2,500 by 0.5. That means 1,250 of your 2,500 calories would come from protein. If you divide those 1,250 calories by 4 (the amount of grams one calorie of protein is equal to), you'll determine that you need 312.5 grams of protein every day. If you eat 7 meals a day and feel you should distribute protein evenly throughout the day, each of those 7 meals would consist of about 45 grams.

If you want 35 percent of the 2,500 calories you've allowed yourself for the day to come from carbohydrates, multiply 2,500 by 0.35. Which means 875 of your 2,500 calories would come from carbohydrates. If you divide those 875 calories by 4 (the amount of grams one calorie of carbohydrate is equal to), you'll determine that you need 218.75 grams of carbohydrates every day. If you eat 7 meals a day and feel you should distribute your carbohydrates evenly throughout the day, each of those 7 meals would consist of about 31 grams.

If you want 15 percent of the 2,500 calories you've allowed yourself for the day to come from fat, multiply 2,500 by 0.15. Which means 375 of your 2,500 calories would come from fat. If you divide those 375 calories by 9 (the amount of grams one calorie of fat is equal to), you'll determine that you need about 42 grams of fat every day. If you eat 7 meals a day and feel you should distribute your fat evenly throughout the day, each of those 7 meals would consist of about 5 grams.

Notice the totals of 45 grams of protein, 31 grams of carbohydrates, and 5 grams of fat that we determined each meal will consist of are very close to the nutritional breakdown of a typical meal replacement shake.

You can check your work by adding the amount of calories you have determined for each of the macronutrients are equal to the daily total of calories for the day in this manner:

Total protein (50%) 1,250
Total carbohydrates (35%) 875
Total fat (15%) 375
Total calories for the day 2,500

Determining your maintenance level

For clarification purposes, your *maintenance* level is the amount of calories you need to stay at your *current* body weight. If you want to gain weight or lose weight, you'll obviously need to make adjustments.

There's really no way of determining *exactly* how many calories you should eat to maintain your current body weight, but here is a method that can get you close to your maintenance level. This method of calculation is called the *Harris-Benedict Equation.* This formula takes into account your sex, age, height, and weight. Other factors are considered as well.

Your heart, breathing, and mental activity all require energy (or calories). Even when you are resting, your body is burning calories to maintain its basic functions. This additional energy requirement is also taken into account by the *Harris-Benedict Equation.*

For men, the equation works as follows: First, multiply your weight by 13.8. Secondly, multiply your height (in inches) by 5. Next, multiply your age by 6.8 then subtract that figure from 67. Add these three totals together.

Here is an example of a 180 pound, 5'9", 23 year-old man:

180 pounds x 13.8 = 2,484.0
69 inches (5'9") x 5 = 345.0
23 years-old x 6.8 = 156.40
67 - 156.4 = - 89.4

Total Calories Needed 2,739.6

For women, the equation works as follows: First, multiply your weight by 9.6. Secondly, multiply your height (in inches) by 1.8. Next, multiply your age by 4.7 then subtract that figure from 65.5. Add these three totals together.

Here is an example of a 120 pound, 5'3", 26 year-old woman:

120 pounds x 9.6 = 1,152.0
63 inches (5'3") x 1.8 = 113.4

26 years-old x 4.7 = 122.2
655 - 122.2 = 532.8

Total Calories Needed 1,798.2

Of course, **this method can only *estimate*** the amount of calories you need to maintain your current weight. You may need to make some adjustments depending on the amount of exercise you do, the type of exercise, and your own individual metabolic factors.

Another way to determine your maintenance level

As I stated earlier, there's really no way of determining *exactly* how many calories you should eat to maintain your current body weight. Here's the challenge. Caloric requirements can change from person to person. Caloric requirements can also change from time period to time period within the same person. You may need to make some adjustments depending on the amount of exercise you do, the type of exercise, and your own individual metabolic factors.

I have a method to make the process of determining the amount of calories you should eat much simpler and probably just as effective.

1. Get a book with a complete listing of foods, their calories, and macronutrient breakdown.

2. Using the information I've provided in the previous section, decide on an appropriate breakdown of macronutrients for your daily food intake. Don't worry about being exact; you can make changes later if necessary.

3. Decide on the number of meals you are committed to eating each day.

4. This may sound too simple, but just pick a total number of calories you'll eat each day and divide that number by the number of meals you are committed to eating. This will give you the total number of calories you should plan to eat during each meal. After determining the amount of calories you should eat each meal, get your complete book of foods and plan your meals from there. 1500, 2000, 3000—whichever number you choose, you'll soon be able to figure out what adjustments you need to make.

<u>**Blood sugar and insulin**</u>

The Doctor Says:
Insulin is the second most powerful hormone in the body behind testosterone when it comes to achieving your bodybuilding goals.

Insulin release is mainly a bodily response, caused by the food you eat. You are able to control this factor to a pretty large degree, just like you can control whether or not you get goose-bumps by making sure to wear a sweater when it's cold; even though the goose-bumps in and by themselves isn't something you can control. You can't choose to have high or low levels of insulin floating around in your system, but you can pretty much steer it by eating. A truckload of fast carbs like Dextrose, a big bowl of rice, and an extended period without food will all have very different impact on your Insulin levels. But let's not rush ahead of ourselves here; let's get the big picture together.

Fast vs. slow burning carbs

As you probably know, carbs are actually plain sugar. As an experiment, chew on a piece of non-sweet bread for a while, and you will notice an increasing sweetness developing, because your saliva and jaw-action is breaking down the large chunks of sugar into smaller units, which in turn gets noticeable as they get smaller and smaller. This is how it works in your stomach as well. Now, the difference between slow and fast carbs, or complex and simple carbs, is how big the chunks of sugar are!

Assume that you have a handful of loose powder. In your stomach, there's really not anything more to digest, so the whole bunch gets launched into the blood stream, which the whole point of eating in the first place, but in this case it all gets launched at the same time, causing a huge, sudden surge of blood sugar! Complex carbs, on the other hand, is more like having a ball of yarn in your hand; it won't just "come apart" anytime soon, but needs to be stripped little by little. This equals a nice and even release of sugar into your blood stream.

Insulin to the rescue

Now, what's the big deal about how fast it goes into the blood stream you may ask? Well, as a general rule, all sudden changes involving the body are bad. The body takes a beating from extreme levels of blood sugar, so in order to protect itself the body releases it's first, last, and only defense against the scum of the blood stream, insulin!

Mr. Insulin is an efficient fellow, rapidly stomping down the blood sugar and thereby saving the body. The bad news is that he's a wee bit over ambitious about it, and usually slashes it down to a level below where it was before eating the food. Now, if you were tired and had low blood sugar before, where do you think you end up half an hour after that candy bar, when Mr. Insulin has done his thing? That's right, a nose dive crash in your energy.

How does insulin work?

Insulin basically force-feeds the muscles with the excess sugar, which they don't like. The amount of sugar being let into the muscles depends on the level of insulin released, which in turn is determined by the insulin receptors in the muscles themselves. Think of it as a person who listens to how hard Mr. Insulin knocks on the door to determine how wide he should open the door. Another feature of insulin is that it is highly anabolic; it's a good friend and ally.

The bad news is that it automatically shuts down your fat burn capacity and keeps it in low gear for quite a while, while actually promoting fat storage! The logic behind this is pretty simple if you remember why insulin is out there in the first place: With this massive dose of sugar going out into the blood, the body makes the assumption that it's getting a truckload of food. Before the days of processed food, it was hard to achieve this kind of sugar-boost without extreme eating, so it makes sense.

What the body does and why

By now one would think that the body would recognize its mistake pretty quickly and correct itself, but this is the part where you sort of get it in the shorts; it won't! At least not for a while. So, to sum it up, you get a sudden blast of sugar in your system, and insulin is released to protect you from it. Mr. Insulin grabs all the sugar and shoves it into the muscles (who don't like it in such high volumes), shuts off the fat burn-switch, and turns on the fat storage-switch.

But since what the body thought was a major load of food really turned out to be only a little candy bar, there is no surplus to handle after that initial blast of sugar ended, so you end up with an empty stomach and even lower blood sugar levels. Normally the body would compensate for this by tapping some stored fat, but the ever-helpful Mr. Insulin made sure to turn that switch off, so what does the body have left? Protein. **More specifically - muscle protein.**

Muscle protein can be used as emergency fuel, especially in a situation where the body perceives itself as starving. Then it wants to get rid of tissue that burns calories 24/7, which leaves us with muscle, being most "un-economical" from a calorie standpoint. It might seem paradoxical about the body both thinking it starves at the same time as it shuts off its fat burn because of anticipated truckloads of food. It is, but there's nothing you can do about it.

Why is insulin so important to me?

For one thing, insulin is an extremely important protector against yourself. If you didn't have insulin to kick in when you got your blood sugar up to dangerous levels, you probably wouldn't live very long. Secondly, it is highly anabolic, and is one of the key factors determining your muscle growth. In this case you're getting some of the bad with the good; you gain overall weight, as in some muscle, some fat. Moderate insulin-levels are beneficial for muscle growth, as long as you don't go overboard.

Stick with pasta, rice, potatoes, oatmeal, and other classic bodybuilding sources of carbs, and you'll probably hit the mark pretty well. You may have noticed that I use fairly negative terms about the insulin force-feeding the muscles with sugar. This is on purpose, simply because it is not a really nice thing to do. I like to compare it to blowing air into lungs that are already full. How would you like that?

Now, the risk here is that the receptors in the muscles, decide that the insulin has been knocking just a little bit too frequently lately, and decides not to open the door as much as it used to. After all, the muscle is not a happy camper about the whole thing in the first place. This is not a concern to the insulin-regulation though, as the primary goal is to get rid of the dangerous sugar from the blood. **So in order to get the job done, more insulin is released to reinforce the effect.** This makes the receptors even more numb, and down the spiral you go. If you keep abusing your body like this, you might end up with **Type II diabetes, where the receptors simply no longer care about the insulin knocking on the door.** The bad news is that decreased insulin sensitivity in the muscles doesn't necessarily mean decreased fat storage capacity, which can be kind of nasty if you have truckloads of insulin floating around.

The Doctor Says:
I don't mean to scare you with the Type II diabetes comment, but just be aware of what foods you are eating and what response they produce once they are in your blood stream.

Keeping your receptors happy and productive

The best way to keep the receptors, and yourself, trim is simple: Train, and cut the fast carbs as much as possible. By training, you deplete the stored carbs in the muscle, so when sugar enters the bloodstream, you're not force feeding the muscles, **you're just feeding them something they want and need!** This is why there's the one exception to the rule about fast carbs: Immediately after training it's good to have something sugary! This is the one time when there's no insulin spike. Why is that? Think of cause and effect; when the muscles were full, they needed to be force-fed more. If they're empty, there's no need to force anything.

Another thing worth mentioning is that **chromium picolinate** can make the receptors more sensitive to insulin, so that less insulin gets the job done. The advantage is obvious: If it'd normally take X amount of insulin to get the job done, that'd result in a certain increase in fat storage. If we cut X by a number of percent, and still get the job done, we automatically cut the increase in fat storage as well! A word of warning though: **This is a long-term effect,** and it's hardly any "miracle pill". Overdosing on chromium will most likely make you more sick than ripped. Keep it sane.

Last but not least, why are we told to take **creatine monohydrate** with something sugary? I'll put it simple: Fast carbs such as sugar; get shoved into the muscles, pronto. Creatine piggybacks on the sugar, and gets shoved into the muscles as well. This makes the creatine absorbed quickly and effectively. For the sake of your health, **I strongly recommend timing this with the post-workout sugar load you have to "refuel" your muscles.** The one time without an insulin-spike, remember?

Insulin summary

- **Eat complex carbs**
- **Avoid simple carbs, except immediately after training**
- **Have your creatine with your post-workout sugar**
- **Take your vitamin/mineral pill every morning**

Now that you've figured out approximately how many calories will maintain your current body weight, all you need to do is eat *less* than that number to lose weight in body fat and eat *more* to gain muscle, right?

Well, it's not that simple. What's most important in building an awesome physique is your *body composition*; not how much you weigh on the scale. Body composition is the makeup of the body in terms of the relative percentage of *lean body mass* and *body fat*. Obviously, having a higher percentage of lean mass and a lower percentage of body fat is ideal. **Your body composition cannot be determined by how much you weigh on a scale.** Changing your eating habits and exercising more can greatly improve your body composition.

When you begin healthier eating habits, be more concerned with the way you *look* and *feel* rather than the bathroom scale. One thing is certain: The scale is not a good indicator if you are adding high-quality muscle mass. The scale can't evaluate how the quality of your training and nutritional habits are affecting your body composition.

You may mistakenly believe an increase in weight is due to more quality muscle and it may be mostly body fat. On the other hand, I have seen quite a few bodybuilders who have obviously gained a fair amount of muscle and, at the same time, lost a considerable amount of body fat, but they were disappointed because they weren't gaining weight.

The best way to monitor your progress is with a mirror. Let me ask you a couple of questions. If you really didn't feel good about the way you looked in the mirror, would a low body fat percentage reading all of a sudden make you happy? In other words, would a "good" number change the vision you see when you look at yourself in the mirror? And, if you we sincerely satisfied with the physique you saw in the mirror, and you were measured at a body fat level higher than you expected, would it change the way you saw yourself? If you answered no to these questions, why would you waste your time getting your body fat levels measured in the first place?

Once again, let the mirror be your guide. Be sure to see what you look like from the rear too! Most of your excess body fat will be carried in your buttocks and hamstrings. What you *can't* see may hurt you!

Build muscle

Eating to build muscle mass

When eating to gain muscle, the best (and the simplest) advice I have ever received was, "Don't eat to get fat. Don't eat to stay lean. Eat to grow!"

Many bodybuilders are confused when it comes to eating the right amount of food necessary to build quality muscle. I suggest starting with the number that you've calculated with the *Harris-Benedict* equation then make adjustments from there.

You often hear about bodybuilders who eat up to 10,000 calories a day. That's a lot of food! No matter how huge you are, that is too much food for your body to digest and use efficiently. At my bodyweight of 200-210 lbs, my calories normally range from 2,500 to 3,200 calories a day.

The Doctor Says:
A good starting point to determine your caloric intake is to divide your calories into protein, carb and fat percentages. Start with 50% of your calories from protein, 35% from carbs and the remaining 15% from fats.

Do you want to make determining the amount of calories you should eat to build muscle and maintain low body fat levels even easier? Just pick a number for your total daily calorie intake like 2,000, 2,500, or 3,000. Then, divide those calories into around 50 percent protein, 35 percent carbohydrates, and 15 percent fat. Use that as a starting point and make adjustments from there.

The bulking up strategy for packing on muscle

Is it better to bulk up for added muscle growth, or stay lean all year around? Unfortunately, this is an area where there are no definitive answers.

One school of thought is that if you consistently ingest high-quality protein and train heavily and efficiently, it is not necessary to put on excess weight to gain muscle. The additional body fat does not pack on more muscle. The more fat you put on, the harder you need to work to melt it off when you want to get lean. This way of thinking advises you to **stay within 10 -15 pounds of your lean, healthy weight** or your shredded contest condition.

I, myself, agree with this thought process. Heavy training, adequate recuperation, and consistently eating high-quality protein are what build rock-solid muscle mass; not excess body fat. The only things extra food and excess body fat can do for you is prevent your body from ever using precious muscle as an energy source, giving you the feeling you have more energy and can train heavier in the gym.

Those are some decent benefits, mind you, but if you are dedicated to be the best bodybuilder you can be, you can get the same benefits by eating smaller, well-balanced meals consistently throughout the day and becoming more focused and mentally tough when you're in the gym.

While I feel certain about my contradicting philosophy, others feel that if you limit the amount of weight you can gain, you will also limit the amount of muscle you can gain in the process. **The trade off is maximum muscle growth with some additional fat or near maximum muscle growth without adding bodyfat.**

If you do decide to bulk up, be sure not to get too far away from contest shape. The longer body fat stays on your body the harder it will be to take it off later. If you get behind schedule and need to drastically reduce your calorie intake to be ready for your contest in time, you will undoubtedly sacrifice a lot of precious muscle in the process. This will negate the very reason why you bulked up in the first place! If you are a drug-free bodybuilder, you do not have any chemicals to help you save muscle. You'll need to use intelligence and discipline.

Whether or not you are a competitive bodybuilder, ultimately you will need to decide how much body fat you are comfortable carrying. It may not be worth it to feel "sloppy" most of the year just to display more muscle on that one day of the contest.

Doctor's Prescription:
Eat to gain muscle, not to get fat. Put on lean bodyweight not sloppy weight. This is even more important if you are involved in any type of sports.

A good rule of thumb when it comes to eating in the off-season is "eat to gain muscle." Do not eat to get fat or eat to stay lean. Consistently feed yourself high-quality protein for muscle growth and enough carbohydrates to keep you feeling your strongest. After prioritizing those needs, consume as much fat as you feel comfortable eating.

How do you know that you're losing muscle?

Some bodybuilders feel if they diet for an extended period of time, they will lose quality muscle. First of all, how do you know you're losing muscle? Are you really lean enough to really tell? Are you sure the size you are losing isn't a lot of water or worthless body fat? Are you sure you just don't look "flat" because your muscles are not filled with glycogen?

Losing muscle just because you are reducing your caloric intake does not have to happen, if you go about it intelligently! It all starts at the dinner table. **You don't need extra carbohydrates or fat in your diet to build or maintain muscle. What you need to build muscle mass is high-quality protein!** Be sure to consume enough of that protein, distribute protein evenly throughout the day, and eat protein often, 6 to 8 times a day.

Doctor's Prescription:
The sure fire way to keep your muscle mass while dieting to lose bodyfat is to keep your protein intake at the same level it has always been. Cut down on the carbs and fats to lower your caloric intake but leave your protein intake the same.

In the gym, you need to train with heavy weight and train with intensity. Then you need to fully recover the muscle before blasting it again and again, week after week.

Like I've said before, the rest is in God's hands. You can, however, make sure you take full responsibility for your part of the muscle-building process. Just make sure you do your part and rest assured that God and Mother Nature will take care of the rest.

Lose fat

Eating to lose body fat

One pound of body fat contains about 3,500 stored calories. You must reduce your caloric intake by 3,500 calories a week to lose one pound per week or increase your activity level to burn 3,500 extra calories per week. **You must either eat fewer calories or burn more calories by increasing your activity level or a combination of both—it's that simple.**

But don't expect getting lean, ripped, or shredded to be so easy. The first few days on a diet, you may lose several pounds. That's because your body takes the easy way out when it needs energy. It uses up your stored carbohydrate (glycogen). Carbohydrates contain a relatively large amount of water. When you begin a diet, you can lose a lot of fluid, but no fat. You have a weight loss that only lasts until your next drink of water.

Your body does other things to preserve body fat. When it has used up its carbohydrate stores, it will shift your metabolism into a slower rate. You will discover you are moving more slowly and have less energy because you have used up your carbohydrate (quick energy) stores. **Our bodies have been conditioned, over time, to guard against famine and will do almost anything to conserve fat.** If weight loss is not done properly, too much precious muscle mass will be lost. But, if you are persistent, as a last resort, your body will begin to use its fat stores for energy.

Don't look too long for easy answers when trying to lose body fat. You are going to have to pay a price if you are truly committed to getting lean. There are no fancy pain-free diets or state-of-the-art supplements that are going to do the bulk of the work for you. Don't try to fool yourself. Or you will set yourself up for failure and disappointment.

The Doctor Says:
There are only 3 major ways to lose weight (preferably bodyfat). Eat less calories, burn more calories or a combination of the two.

If you want to lose excess body fat, the bottom line is you have to eat fewer calories than you burn each day. There are several ways to burn more calories than you eat. You can add more cardiovascular work to your training regimen. You can also simply eat less food throughout the day. You can even do a combination of these two strategies by doing more cardiovascular training and eating less food.

How quickly you will shred that body fat will depend on how much of a deficit you create between the calories you consume and the calories you burn on a daily basis. And for how long you wish to go through the sacrifice and pain it takes to train and/or diet this way.

Although my advice doesn't make the fat loss process a whole lot easier, it should make the process simpler. Without being distracted by constantly searching for unrealistic, quick fix solutions, or super supplements. You can now focus on the task in front of you, get to work and achieve the results you truly desire.

Here is an example breakdown of how a 200 pound bodybuilder can gain/maintain muscle while dropping bodyfat. It will give you 300 grams of carbs and 200 grams of protein.

Meal one: Breakfast

75-100 grams of carbs

35 grams of protein

Meal two: Mid-morning snack

25 grams of carbs

25 grams of protein

Meal three: Lunch

50 grams of carbs

35 grams of protein

Meal four: Postworkout

75-100 grams of carbs

55 grams of protein

Meal five: Dinner

50 grams of carbs

35 grams of protein

Meal six: Bedtime snack

No carbs

25 grams of protein

There's no substitute for hard work when it comes to losing fat

When it comes to dieting to lose bodyfat, there's no substitute for hard work. Believe me, I really wish this were not the case. If it really was that easy then everyone would have already done it and we would live in a world of perfect bodies! Unfortunately, however, you must burn more calories than you ingest every day to lose that stubborn body fat.

Low-fat diets, high fat diets, carefully watching your fat intake, or paying close attention to the glycemic index in your foods, it doesn't matter. When the day is done, you must burn more calories than you eat. It doesn't even matter if all the food you eat is healthy, non-junk food, or "clean," its total must be lower than your maintenance level.

As the saying goes, "God puts a price-tag on everything." If you've accumulated some body fat and desperately want to get rid of it, you are going to have to pay the price. The price may be spending more time sweating on a treadmill, feeling hungry on occasion, or both. Whatever method you choose, there will be some pain involved. I would be lying to you if I told you any differently.

Anyone who tells you differently is just flat-out misleading you! I firmly believe it is our desire to discover some painless alternative that we mistakenly believe is "somewhere out there" which prevents us from dieting the way we must in order to accomplish our goal of losing body fat.

There are several ways to burn more calories than you eat. You can add more cardiovascular work to your training regimen, simply eat less food throughout the day, or even do a combination of more cardiovascular training and eating less food.

Can I build muscle and lose fat at the same time?

One question I am continually asked is, "Is it possible to lose body fat and gain muscle at the same time?" My answer is an emphatic yes!

First of all, to build muscle, you must constantly overload the muscles in the gym. Heavy training is of utmost importance. Even when you are on a calorie-deprived diet to lose body fat, you must be mentally tough and continue to train heavily to preserve and even build muscle mass. And, as I've discussed several times already, back up heavy training by eating high-quality protein on a consistent basis.

To lose body fat and still gain muscle, you must really watch your diet closely. Keep your daily caloric intake below your maintenance level. When you reduce your calories, be sure to keep your diet high in quality protein. **Most of your calories should come from your protein consumption.** Of course, watch your fat intake.

The Doctor Says:
Building muscle and losing bodyfat at the same time is a process that is a natural defense mechanism for the body. Don't let others mislead you when they say it can't be done, they just don't know all the facts.

Here is how I suggest you manipulate your carbohydrate consumption: For a couple of days, eat only vegetables for carbohydrates then go back to grains like rice, potatoes, and pasta for a couple of days. Rotate in this manner and see how quickly you start melting the fat. Because carbohydrates give you energy, this may become difficult at times. Nevertheless, it is a very effective strategy.

Getting shredded and keeping mass

I believe getting ripped is a matter of having a little bit of knowledge, but most important, having a lot of "heart". It takes a lot of discipline to stay on your diet for a longer time than others who have faster metabolisms or who use chemicals to assist them.

You have to go hungry sometimes while continuing to train hard and heavy so you can retain as much muscle as possible. I believe many more drug-free bodybuilders could be in better condition. **It is a matter of whether or not they are willing to do the hard work and go through the sacrifice that's required.**

Fat-burning mode: learn to love it

Over the years, I've learned to become acute to my body's signals that let me know if I'm on the right track to gradually lose fat. I can tell when I am turning my body into a "fat-burning machine" or in other words, when I feel as though my body is running at an optimal fat-burning mode. What does that feel like? Well, for starters, I have that "hungry-but-not-hungry feeling" most of the time. My stomach never feels full, even immediately after eating a meal. The most I ever feel is satisfied. My body temperature is much hotter throughout the day and I am sweating more profusely during my cardiovascular sessions.

The Doctor Says:
When you get in touch with your body you can actually "feel" that your body is in fat burn mode. Not that you can feel the fat cells being depleted but there are other cues that tell you the process is occurring.

Many bodybuilders get "freaked out" when they see what their body looks like when it's in fat-burning mode. They fear that they are getting small and losing muscle. Visually, my body does appear to be smaller and my clothes fit more loosely. My muscle-bellies are much flatter than when I'm eating more food. It's not that I'm losing muscle; it's just that my muscles are not filled with as much glycogen, therefore look like deflated balloons. This is a necessary evil; at least for a period of time.

I have learned over the years to associate positive emotions to these kinesthetic-external and visual feelings during the dieting process, not fear. These are sure-fire indicators that I am well on my way to being in the shape I want and the look that I am going for.

Top 8 fitness success formulas

If there's one thing we've learned by now, it's that the drastic, cut out all (carbs, fat, protein, sugar, dairy, eggs, calories heck - why not everything?) Diets are not the answer to the energy and physique you want. Sure, you're going to drop some pounds pretty fast, but they're unlikely to stay away very long.

Now, there are two schools of thought when it comes to making major changes in your life. Some experts agree that making small changes in your diet and activity level will add up to a slow and steady weight loss. And the simpler they are, the more likely you'll stick with them for the rest of your life.

These experts reason that if you make a really dramatic change, you'll be so overwhelmed that you'll just go back to what you were doing before. Sounds good, doesn't it? It's like they're saying, "You can still make changes, but you don't have to get out of your comfort zone to do it."

Here's the deal: while we generally know what to do and how to do it, there needs to be a catalyst of some sort to ignite the change process. But doing something you're used to doing will keep getting you the results you've been getting.

Massive action, man. Get out of that comfort zone. DO IT.

Be confident and take BIG steps to change. Create momentum for yourself so that you become unstoppable. Having a leaner, energized, body with confidence and determination is important to you, SO GO GET IT. Let others know what you're doing to give yourself more leverage to keep at it.

The math is simple. To lose a pound of fat you need to burn 3500 more calories than you take in. So if you burn 200 calories from working out and shave 300 calories from what you normally eat in a day, you'll lose that pound of fat.

If you want to lose 1.5 pounds of fat, bump up the intensity of your exercise. I don't recommend cutting your calories drastically, since you need to feed your body nourishing food for it to perform at its best, protect muscle, have energy, and mental performance.

So if you burn an extra 250 calories on top of the 200 you're already burning (and it's easy to do), you can lose the 1.5 pounds of fat. A 30-minute strength training workout can incinerate 200-500 calories. Compliment it with aerobics, and you're on your way to melting off 12 pounds of ugly fat in about two months.

Take a look at this list of seven mini-recipes for your health and fitness success. DO THEM. If they're not working for you, re-word them so that they do. The goal is to simplify the success process.

1. Listen to your body

Are you truly hungry when you eat, or do you end to snack out of habit without paying attention to your appetite? If you're eating when you're not hungry, those are usually extra calories that your body doesn't need.

So, before you reach for a snack, ask yourself if you're physically hungry. Sometimes hunger is a sign of thirst, so try drinking a big glass of water and see if your appetite subsides. If you are physically hungry, eat a nutritious, balanced snack.

FORMULAS:
STOP + ASK = SAVE CALORIES
STOP/ASK + DRINK WATER = CONTROL APPETITE

2. Control your portions

Many of us tend to eat more serving of low-fat or fat-free foods like bread, bagels, cereals, and desserts than we realize. We hear too much about cutting out the fat, but not enough of "control your portions."

Check the labels to compare its portion size to what you're really eating. You may be in for an eye-opener. A half-cup of pasta is about 200 calories, so a plateful of pasta could end up being some 600 calories, NOT including sauce, bread, and meat or protein source. Wow. Now you're talking a potential 1000 calorie dinner.

Then there's the "dining out challenge." Look, you don't HAVE to eat what they've served you. Eat maybe a third of what's on your plate, then bring the rest home. That way you'll still feel satisfied.

You also don't have to measure your portions. Use the palm of your hand as a measuring device. The "eyeball method," I call it. For veggies, fill 2-3 palmsful for a serving; fruits, 1 palmful; protein, 1 palmful; and fat, the round line around your thumb area (about 1-2 tsp.)

FORMULAS:
CHECK LABEL + STICK WITH THAT SERVING SIZE = SAVE CALORIES
DINE OUT + CUT PORTIONS BY 1/3 = CUT CALORIES
EYEBALL METHOD + BALANCE MEALS = MORE NUTRITION WITH LESS CALORIES

3. Slow down!

If you're a fast eater, try these two tips for helping you eat less and still feel satisfied:

1. At the beginning of your meal, eat something you can't consume quickly, like hot soup or spicy salsa. If you're forced to slow down, you'll give your body a chance to feel satisfied before you overeat.

2. Put your fork or spoon down in between bites, and keep the TV or radio off. It takes about 20 minutes for you to feel full, so take time to enjoy your food instead of scarfing it down.

FORMULAS:
"SPEED BUMP" FOOD + SLOW DOWN = SATISFACTION WITHOUT OVEREATING
PUT FORK/SPOON DOWN + QUIET SETTING = ENJOY FOOD & FEEL SATISFIED

4. Substitute smarter

Look at foods you regularly eat and try to cut calories that you won't miss. For instance, if you always eat a scrambled egg with breakfast, scramble two egg whites. Or substitute mustard for mayonnaise on your sandwich. Try the new Pam cooking sprays that are butter, olive, or garlic flavored on your cooked veggies instead of butter.

FORMULA:
FOOD + SUBSTITUTE = CUT CALORIES WITHOUT CUTTING FLAVOR

5. What are you drinking?

If you regularly down lattes, cafe mochas, or sweetened beverages, you're drinking more calories than you realize. Research has shown that people don't think of beverages as food. If you have a couple of glasses of orange juice for breakfast, that's at least 300 calories right there.

Cutting back on coffee and tea can have a marked improvement on your weight if you normally add cream and sugar. Little things make a huge difference.

FORMULAS:

NORMAL BEVERAGE + DRINK STRAIGHT = SAVE CALORIES
ATTITUDE ABOUT DRINK + SUBSTITUTE OR ELIMINATE = CUT CALORIES

6. Get your butt in gear

Of course you knew I was going to mention exercise at some point in this article. You just can't overlook the calorie-burning benefits of exercise. Now exercise is not just about aerobics and lifting weights. You can burn a good amount of calories by doing housework or yard work with some vigor. Remember, LITTLE THINGS... Also remember, LIFE IS EXERCISE. So shoot for 30 minutes each day.

FORMULA:
EXERCISE + DAILY = SERIOUS CALORIE BURNING

7. Join your kids

Just because you're running around with your kids with their activities doesn't mean you can't be active yourself. Going to your kid's soccer game? Walk around the field while you're watching.

Get them involved with physical fitness. If your kids are old enough, make it a family-thing to go for a walk together, or a bike ride. If you're watching TV, make it a game and see how many push ups each of you can do during commercials (or crunches) before the show comes back on.

FORMULA:
FAMILY + ACTIVITY = EXTRA CALORIE BURNING AND FIT FAMILY
KIDS' ACTIVITIES + ACTIVE WATCHING ACTIVITY = NO EXCUSE FOR "NO TIME"

8. Build muscle!

If you want to achieve lasting weight loss, be SURE to include strength training into your fitness routine. You know the story: lean muscle increases your metabolism, allowing you to burn more calories even at rest; you're stronger, so you fatigue less often and not as quickly; you melt off fat faster, so you can sculpt a great looking body.

FORMULAS:
STRENGTH TRAINING + METABOLISM = LASTING WEIGHT LOSS
STRENGTH TRAINING + PROPER NUTRITION = HIGH METABOLISM
STRENGTH TRAINING + AEROBIC CONDITIONING = ENERGY, VITALITY, BODY YOU WANT

Work with your metabolism

Dealing with a slow metabolism

Many people are confused and frustrated about what they can do to reach their physique goals—despite having a slow metabolism. My suggestions for dealing with a slow metabolism are two-fold: First, there are a few procedures that you can follow to help your metabolism run more efficiently. Secondly, conquering the challenge of a slow metabolism by changing the way you look at it.

Procedures you can implement to speed up your metabolism:

1. Obviously, **consuming fewer calories will speed up your metabolism.** Your body must work harder with less fuel to train in the gym and accomplish your other daily activities. As long as you keep what you believe to be the proper ratio of protein, carbohydrates and fat for your body, it will run more efficiently with less food for a while.

2. **Rotate the amount of calories you eat.** Your body will eventually adapt to the amount of calories you ingest and slow down in it's effort to hold onto and store body fat. If you feel your body burns about 2,500 calories a day, eat only 2,000 for a few days. Then, go back to eating 2,500 for a stretch of days. Again, for a few days, eat only 2,000. Then, to really keep your body from adapting and slowing down your metabolism, eat 3,000 for a few days. Continue rotating your caloric intake in this manner.

3. Eat smaller, more frequent meals throughout the day.

4. Cut down on starchy carbohydrates and, of course, your fat intake.

5. Replace most of your carbohydrate calories with "good" fats like canola oil or olive oil. Make sure you replace an equal amount of carbohydrate calories with fat calories. Fat, when added to your diet in this type of manner, becomes a much more efficient source of energy for the body to use.

6. Try eating only fibrous, vegetable carbohydrates for a series of days.

7. Increase your cardiovascular training.

8. Try doing your cardiovascular training first thing in the morning before you eat breakfast.

9. Consider taking a thermogenic, fat-burning, metabolism-increasing supplement.

Mental strategies for dealing with a slow metabolism

The mental aspect of overcoming this obstacle is what I'll now address. When you've labeled your metabolism as "slow," with whom or what are you comparing? A 73 year-old woman? A 19 year-old guy in your gym? How efficiently your body ran 15 years ago?

Why waste your energy lamenting about the fast metabolism you had in days gone by? Why waste time comparing yourself with those who have faster metabolisms? Why spend any of your precious time "cursing the Gods above" for being put in such a challenging position?

But you know what? Who cares? If I'm truly committed to getting shredded, I'll make the required adjustments. I must create a significant deficit from the amount of calories I consume versus the amount of calories my body actually burns each day, whatever those numbers are. The bottom line is that I need to either eat fewer calories, do more cardiovascular training, or a combination of both. The responsibility is squarely on my own shoulders!

Deal with reality. If you are truly committed to achieving your goals, then make the necessary adjustments based on what you have or don't have. Spend your time and energy striving to be the very best that you can be.

The Doctor Says:
I know it's easy to use the excuse that your slow metabolism is making it impossible to build the body you want. The fact is you have to work with what you have and you can do it because other people just like you have done it. So can you.

Dealing with a fast metabolism

The major challenges a bodybuilder with a fast metabolism compared to a person with an average metabolism is that he must invest additional time, better time management, and more money for extra food. If a person with an average metabolism needs to eat six well-balanced meals spread evenly throughout the day to reach their bodybuilding goals, a person with a fast metabolism may have to eat eight or nine. The body's higher caloric requirement will be satisfied by the additional meals. The type of foods and the proportion of macronutrients that a bodybuilder with a fast metabolism needs to meet their goals are the same as a person with an average one.

<u>Importance of post workout nutrition</u>

Invest your time wisely

You don't need to be a resource management specialist to know that time is the most valuable finite resource that you have. And as you well know, there's a very limited amount of it to go around. So if you're smart, you'll figure out ways to get the greatest return on the investment of your time.

While this may be well recognized and applied in many aspects of modern life, it confuses me as to why people seem to ignore this when it comes to their exercise training. From what I see on a daily basis, it's clear to me that most people in the gym are wasting their time investment. They're spending precious hours engaged in strength or endurance training programs that yield little or no results?

Need proof? When was the last time someone in your gym made any noticeable physical progress? In fact, when was the last time that you made any significant physical progress? Exercise training has the potential to yield huge returns on any given time investment. Isn't it a shame that most people don't ever see this magnitude of return?

The Doctor Says:
I know I sound like a motivational speaker or a financial planner when I say this but you do need to use your time to your advantage. The proper use of your time is the single biggest factor whether you will be a success or failure in life.

Despite this disappointing reality, I'm here to tell you that hope is not lost. In fact, there's a very easy way to capitalize on your investment. You see, in most cases the exercise is not the problem. The problem is that people fail to invest in the other important commodity that, in combination with exercise, yields the biggest returns.

They're buying the cart without the horse, the lemonade stand without the lemonade. They're spending their time focused on only the exercise program while ignoring the importance of a sound nutritional program.

Now I could write a dozen articles focused on straightening out the nutritional problems of the world. But those articles are for another day. Today I intend to focus on what is, in my opinion, the most important aspect of exercise nutrition; eating during the post-workout period. The knowledge of how to eat during this time will maximize your efforts in the gym and yield the biggest returns on your time investment.

Remodeling the post-workout period

Exercise, both strength and endurance training, are responsible for countless health and aesthetic benefits. However the exercise itself is a significant physiological stressor.

Perceived symptoms of this "stress" are often mild and include muscle soreness, the need for extra sleep, and an increased appetite.

These symptoms let us know that the exercise has depleted the muscle's fuel resources, caused some minor damage, and that the muscle is in need of replenishment and repair. While the words depletion and damage may sound like negative things, they're not if they only stick around for a short period of time. You see, these changes allow the muscle to adapt by getting better at the exercise demands placed on it.

Therefore if you're doing endurance exercise, the muscle will become depleted and damaged in the short run, but in the long run it will super compensate, building itself up to be a better aerobic machine. And if strength training is your thing, you'll tear down you're weaker muscle fibers in favor of building up bigger, stronger ones.

In all cases, exercise essentially tears down old, less adapted muscle in order to rebuild more functional muscle. This phenomenon is called remodeling. While the remodeling process is much more complex than I can describe here, it's important for me to emphasize that this remodeling only takes place if the muscle is provided the right raw materials. If I plan on remodeling my home I can hire a guy to tear down a couple of walls, a guy to clean up the mess, and a guy to come in and rebuild better walls than the ones that came down. But if I don't give that guy any bricks, how's he going to get anything done? If I don't give him the bricks, all I'll have in the end is a much smaller, unfinished house.

The same holds true with exercise remodeling. In particular, during the exercise bout and the time immediately following it, exercise breaks down our muscle carbohydrate stores and our muscle protein structures. Then, the immune system comes in to clean up the mess. And finally, signals are generated to tell the body to rebuild. However, without the proper protein and carbohydrate raw materials, this building can't take place. You'll be left with muscles that never reach their potential.

So with this analogy, I hope it's obvious that this post-exercise period is not a time to take lightly. Remember, you spent a significant amount of time in the gym breaking down the muscle for a good reason. You want it to be better adapted to future demands. So to realize full return on your time investment, you need to give the body the raw materials it needs, namely protein and carbohydrates.

You have to feed your hungry muscles

As I mentioned, all trainees (male or female), regardless of their chosen mode of exercise, must take their post-exercise nutrition seriously in order to provide the muscle with the raw materials it needs. As all types of exercise use carbohydrates for energy, muscle carbohydrate depletion is inevitable. Therefore a post-workout meal high in carbohydrates is required to refill muscle carbohydrate/energy stores.

However any ol' amount of carbohydrates will not do. You need to consume enough carbohydrates to promote a substantial insulin release. **Insulin is the hormone responsible for shuttling carbohydrates and amino acids into the muscle.** In doing this, carbohydrate re-synthesis is accelerated and protein balance becomes positive, leading to rapid repair of the muscle tissue.

Therefore, **by consuming a large amount of carbohydrates, you will promote a large insulin release, increase glycogen storage, and increase protein repair.** Research has shown that a carbohydrate intake of 0.8 to 1.2 grams per 1 kilogram of body weight, for your post workout meal, maximizes glycogen synthesis and accelerates protein repair. However, unless you've had a very long, intense workout, 1.2g/kg may be a bit excessive as excess carbohydrate can be converted to bodyfat. Therefore I recommend 0.9g of carbohydrate per 1 kilogram of body weight for speeding up muscle carbohydrate replenishment while preventing excess fat gain.

In addition, since muscle protein is degraded during exercise, the addition of a relatively large amount of protein to your post exercise meal is necessary to help rebuild the structural aspects of the muscle. After exercise, the body decreases its rate of protein synthesis and increases its rate of protein breakdown. However, the provision of protein and amino acid solutions has been shown to reverse this trend, increasing protein synthesis and decreasing protein breakdown.

Researchers have used anywhere from 0.2g - 0.4g of protein per 1 kilogram of body weight to demonstrate the effectiveness of adding protein to a post-workout carbohydrate drink. As an increased consumption of the essential amino acids may lead to a more positive protein balance, 0.4g/kg may be better than 0.2g/kg.

While your post-workout feeding should be rich protein and carbohydrate, this meal should be fat free. The consumption of essential fats is one of the most overlooked areas of daily nutritional intake but during the post workout period, eating fat can actually decrease the effectiveness of your post-workout beverage. Since fat slows down transit through the stomach, eating fat during the post workout period may slow the digestion and absorption of carbohydrates and proteins. As your post workout feeding should be designed to promote the most rapid delivery of carbohydrates and protein to your depleted muscles, fats should be avoided during this time.

Finally, another important factor to consider is the timing of this meal. **It is absolutely crucial that you consume your post-workout meal immediately after exercise.** As indicated above, after exercise, the muscles are depleted and require an abundance of protein and carbohydrate. In addition, during this time, the muscles are biochemically "primed" for nutrient uptake.

This phenomenon is commonly known as the "window of opportunity". Over the course of the recovery period, this window gradually closes and by failing to eat immediately after exercise, you diminish your chances of promoting full recovery. To illustrate how quickly this window closes, research has shown that **consuming a post-exercise meal immediately after working out is superior to consuming one only 1 hour later.** In addition, consuming one 1 hour later is superior to consuming one 3 hours later. If you wait too long, glycogen replenishment and protein repair will be compromised.

So, when you decided to start exercising you decided to give up a specific amount of time per week in the interest of getting better, physically. However, if you haven't spent the necessary time thinking about post-exercise nutrition, you're missing much of the benefit that comes with exercising. I assure you that once you start paying attention to this variable in the recovery equation, your time in the gym will be much better invested. The results you will obtain will be all the proof you need.

Whole food vs. nutritional supplements

Anchored firmly atop their calorie-counting soapbox, nutritionists have traditionally asserted that whole food always trumps supplemental nutrition. For them I have only one sentiment: "Always...it is a meaningless word." -Oscar Wilde

While I wholeheartedly believe that complete, unbleached, untreated, and unprocessed whole food should form the basis of any sound nutritional regimen, there are some instances in which supplements can actually be superior to whole food. In the case of post-exercise nutrition, I believe that liquid supplemental nutrition is far superior to whole food for the following reasons.

Doctor's Prescription:
Use liquid meals (i.e. protein drinks) when it is beneficial to your body and your schedule to do so. Also, filling in some of the snacks in-between your whole food meals with protein drinks is a good way to keep your protein intake spread out.

Liquid meals taste good and are getting better

Typically, after intense exercise, most people complain that eating a big meal is difficult. This is understandable as the exercise stress creates a situation where the hunger centers are all but shut down. However, as you now know, it's absolutely critical that you eat if you want to remodel the muscle, enlarge the muscle, or recover from the exercise.

Fortunately liquid supplemental formulas are palatable, easy to consume, and can be quite nutrient dense, providing all the nutrition you need at this time. In addition, since these formulas are structurally simple; the gastrointestinal tract has no difficulty processing them. **Your stomach will thank you for this.**

Liquid meals have a fast absorption profile

The latest research has demonstrated that liquid supplemental formulas containing fast digesting protein (whey hydrolysates and isolates) and carbohydrates (dextrose and maltodextrin) are absorbed more quickly than whole food meals. To put this into perspective, **a liquid post-exercise formula may be fully absorbed within 30 to 60 minutes**, providing much needed muscle nourishment by this time. However, a slower digesting solid food meal may take 2 to 3 hours to fully reach the muscle.

Liquid meals take advantage of the window of opportunity

The faster the protein and carbohydrates get to the muscle, the better your chances for muscle building and recovery. Speed is of the essence when it comes to using your window of opportunity. Current research has demonstrated that subjects receiving nutrients within one hour after exercise recover more quickly than subjects receiving nutrients three hours after exercise. Liquid nutrition is making more sense, isn't it?

Liquid meals are better for nutrient targeting

During the post exercise period, specific nutrients maximize your recovery. These include an abundance of water, high glycemic index carbohydrates, and certain amino acids. It's also best to avoid fat during this time. So the only way to ensure that these nutrients are present in the right amounts is to formulate a specific liquid blend. Whole foods may miss the mark.

Keep your diet super simple

Have you ever known people who are always asking themselves "What am I going to eat for dinner tonight?" Some people put a lot of thought and effort into deciding what they are going to enjoy for their next meal. In my opinion, they make the eating process far too complicated!

I intentionally keep my meals plain and simple. I don't get too fancy or complicated when it comes to eating. I eat to grow muscle and keep my body fat levels manageable. When you eat the way you need in order to grow and get your momentum rolling, even plain and boring meals can taste delicious; if you have the right mindset and are hungry enough. If you really want anything in life, there is always a price you're going to pay.

I'm not saying everyone should eat the way I do, but if you want to build muscle in the shortest amount of time, this is what I've found to be the most effective route. You can adjust your standards in any way you wish depending on your own physique goals. You must understand I am trying to become the very best I can be at what I do and am trying to share the strategies that have worked for me. I understand there is more than one way to "skin a cat" but this is the system I have chosen.

Food is a vehicle that, if utilized properly, can help me reach my ultimate goals as a bodybuilder and much more. If used improperly, food can hinder, or even destroy, my dreams. Keep this in mind when you are hungry for McDonald's or something. I really don't mind eating the same foods every day. It makes my life simpler so I can concentrate on things in my life that I feel are more important.

Be consistent, always

Bodybuilding is a lifestyle. Doing it correctly does not stop after you are done in the gym. **You must constantly feed your body the right foods if you want to enjoy a great physique.**

Some natural bodybuilders make a terrible mistake of being inconsistent. When they want to prepare for a show, they start "bearing down" two or three months before. This is usually much too late. Some of the best drug-assisted bodybuilders may be able to get by with this habit, but a successful natural bodybuilder cannot.

How you eat seven months before a show is just as important as how you eat seven weeks, or even seven days, before a show. If you wait until three months before, you are losing a lot of precious time that you could use for growing by staying consistent with your nutritional habits.

If you are a non-competitive bodybuilder, consistent eating habits are just as important to you. If you want to feel strong, be strong, and look your best you must **"feed the machine."** Patience is a very important part of your ability to stick to your nutritional program.

Countless benefits to having good nutrition habits

Sound nutrition has many more benefits than just aesthetics. Applying good eating habits to your daily life will also help you mentally. If your body is a machine that needs fuel to run properly, then food is that fuel. The higher quality food you give your machine, the better it will perform. Performing better means a better sense of well being, sharper thinking, more strength in the gym, and better performance in other areas of your life, such as work and relationships with people. I believe when you consistently eat right, you have more "pep in your step," the sky seems a lot bluer, the air seems a lot fresher and you become a happier, more optimistic person.

It goes without saying you will need to put forth some effort — and this can become very difficult. Isn't anything worth having always a little difficult? Attaining a muscular physique you can be proud of is one of these difficult tasks. Eating properly on a consistent basis is going to help you reach your goals.

Sometimes, it doesn't matter how committed, dedicated, or disciplined you are. If you don't have an outstanding strategy, you will not achieve outstanding results. Hard work will only go so far. Hard work may get you in very good condition—but not outstanding.

The Doctor Says:
I could go on and on until I am blue in the face about how important nutrition is but I think you get the picture.

Fat provides a consistent, slow-burning, and extremely efficient source of energy. Carbohydrates are often hot-and-cold and tend to spike your insulin levels. Excess carbohydrates can easily be stored as fat. Keeping your carbohydrates very low while adding good fat to your diet in its place will keep you strong in the gym and keep you looking full. Along with my hard work, eating this way for months enabled my body to melt the extremely-hard-to-burn marbled fat deep within my muscles.

The importance of drinking plenty of water

Water is one of the most precious resources on the planet. All life depends on water. The Earth and everything living thing upon it is primarily made of water. As human beings, **our bodies are over 67 percent water** and need to replenish with plenty of water on a continual basis to function properly. If we do not drink enough water, everything from our cells to our bodily organs and how they function will be compromised.

Your muscles are 70 percent water and it plays a major role in the muscle building process. How exactly does water help build muscle? In general terms, water helps your body properly utilize the nutritious foods you are committed to eating while efficiently eliminating waste.

Drinking plenty of water aids in the digestion of nutrients, how efficiently those nutrients are transported to the cells, and how well the cells absorb them. One of water's most important roles is to flush the dangerous toxins out of our bodies. Every function of the human body will be compromised on a systemic level when you don't drink enough water.

Water helps you get the most value from your supplements as well. Water helps with the utilization of all the water-soluble vitamins and minerals your body needs to survive. If a person is not getting significant results from **creatine, which in my opinion is one the most effective legal supplements of the market,** I would surmise they are not drinking enough water to take advantage of the hydration effect that occurs. In the gym, water helps prevent injuries that may occur during weight training by cushioning joints and other soft tissue areas.

I try to drink almost a gallon of water a day to keep my body healthy and support my bodybuilding efforts. This is the normal amount for a bodybuilder my size; you may need more if you are 230+ lbs. or are on a steroid cycle. This is quite an investment in time, effort, and visits to the bathroom, but I'm certain it is a wise investment. You won't see me anywhere without my plastic jug of water nearby.

My tip for drinking more water. Slightly sweetening your water with Crystal Light will help you get much more down each day. Don't follow the directions for use, however. All of that Crystal Light, although relatively low in calories, will give you too much flavor, which is rather sour. Diluting the Crystal Light tastes much better! I put 1/2 of one of those little "tubs" in every gallon of water I drink. I think that adds about 50 calories for the day, which is well worth the investment!

Doctor's Prescription:
In addition to the plain water you drink, include the natural water that is found in fruits and vegetables to your total water intake each day. For example, I drink almost ¾ gallon of plain water each day and get about ¼ gallon of water from fruits and vegetables.

Having cheat days in your diet without guilt

Always schedule in advance the days that you'll stray or "cheat" from your well-planned and structured bodybuilding diet instead of arbitrarily doing so. You'll feel more successful, in control, and dedicated. You'll become more determined to make it to the "finish line" after you've put together a stretch of days exhibiting outstanding discipline. You will enjoy the "not-so-healthy" meals even more and with less guilt because you know you've earned that indulgence.

Eating out

If you're like most people, you're eating out more than ever. With a little effort, however, you can have almost as much control over what you eat when you dine out as you do at home. The following tips give you the tools you need to win at the restaurant game.

1. **Get a Little Something on the Side.** Salad dressing is not the only topping that can be served on the side. You can make the same request with sour cream, sauces and most seasonings. Unless the dish is pre-made, such as frozen lasagna, having the kitchen omit a sauce or serve a topping separately is perfectly acceptable.

2. **Ask until you're Satisfied.** Perhaps the most effective method of getting what you want in a restaurant is to ask questions. Whether your question is about ingredients, preparation methods, price, portion size or substitutions, don't settle for a half-baked answer. If your server seems unsure of the answer to your question, have him or her ask a manager.

3. **Know When to Go.** If you have special instructions for the kitchen, you may want to eat out during non-peak hours. Between 7:00 and 8:30 pm, most good restaurants get very busy, and your special order may take a little longer; or if you end up having to send it back, a lot longer. Try going before the dinner rush.

4. **Fib a Little.** What's the best way to be sure the oil is left out of your pasta primavera? Tell your server you are allergic to an ingredient in the oil, or you have a dangerous reaction to oil because of a medication you're taking.

5. **Use Threats.** Politely ask your server to tell the kitchen you will send your food back if it's not prepared to your specifications. This ensures the kitchen will make it right the first time. Remember, it's usually the fault of the cook, not the server, if your food is not prepared properly.

6. **Try to Be a Kid Again.** Many restaurants have a special children's section on the menu that you may be able to order from. If not, ask the waiter or the manager, if you may have a half order of something. Managers are usually eager to please.

7. **Don't Be a Softie.** When the dessert cart comes around, don't feel bad about saying, "No, thanks," even if a server pressures you. The same goes for unwanted appetizers, drinks or "extra" side dishes. You will not hurt the server's feelings by saying no.

8. **Stop Eating When You Are Full.** Ask someone, your server, a busboy, a manager or another server to take your plate when you have had enough. If you can see as soon as you get your plate that the portion is too large, as it will be in most restaurants these days, immediately divide the food in half. Put one part in a to-go box or just place it to the side.

9. **Be a Regular.** If you go to the same place often and get to know the staff by name, your requests and questions are more likely to be taken seriously. Who knows, maybe you'll even have a dish named after you!

10. **Tip Generously.** Like it or not, the restaurant business is a service industry where you are the boss. If you take care of your server, he or she will take care of you.

Power up your breakfast

As many of you know, breakfast is the most important meal of the day. It is amazing how many people skip this valuable meal. If you are a bodybuilder or not, breakfast plays a vital role for your metabolism and over all health. Let's just take the time to look at the word itself, "Break-Fast". That is essentially what we are doing in the morning when we eat. We are breaking the fast our bodies go through from our last meal the night before, through the 8 to 10 hours of sleep we get a night.

During your sleep time

During the night, especially for body builders, your nitrogen balance fluctuates from a positive balance into a negative nitrogen balance. Nitrogen balance is when a person's daily intake of nitrogen from proteins equals the daily excretion of nitrogen. A negative nitrogen balance occurs when the excretion of nitrogen exceeds the daily intake and is often seen when muscle is being lost. On the other end of the spectrum, a positive nitrogen balance is often associated with muscle growth. In other words our metabolisms turn catabolic (breakdown of muscle tissue for energy metabolism) during sleep, a condition no bodybuilder wants to be in if he/she desires maximum muscle growth.

What happens is your hard-earned muscle tissue is robbed of important amino acids to be synthesized into glucose to fuel the brain, nervous system, and other organs and tissues. Don't panic, this is a natural process our bodies go through to sustain life every day. Our goal is to keep the state of negative nitrogen balance to a minimum and throw that balance into a positive through diet and nutrition and by making sure we eat a well-balanced breakfast.

This however should definitely assure you to think twice before skipping breakfast. Breakfast feeds your body the fuel it is in need for and serves to jumpstart and speed up the metabolism. **Just by eating breakfast, containing all of the three main components (protein, carbs, and fat) can raise your metabolism 60-100%.** So with this in mind it would sound foolish to even think about skipping the most important meal of the day.

Doctor's Prescription:
Have breakfast everyday and make sure you have some protein in your breakfast too. If you are like me, I know you have very little time first thing in the morning but make breakfast your priority.

This will take you out of the negative nitrogen balance (catabolism, breakdown of protein), and hopefully switch you into a positive nitrogen balance (Anabolism: process of building up complex materials, proteins, from simple materials). Positive nitrogen balance is the environment you want to be in to promote lean muscle mass and accelerated fat loss.

O.K., now that we know the importance of breakfast for your health, metabolism, and fitness gains, we now need to know what to eat for breakfast. A lot of people think a bowl of hot cereal and a piece of fruit is a nutritious breakfast. Guess again! Yes these are healthy choices, but the meal is incomplete. Breakfast, along with the rest of your meals, should contain a balance of protein, complex carbohydrates, and fats (fats usually occur naturally and do not have to be added). I'll give you an analogy.

Your car needs water, oil, and gas to run efficiently. If you leave one of those three properties out, your car is not going to run. The same goes for our bodies. We must include all three nutrients, especially protein and high-fiber complex carbohydrates, to function at peak performance and to get all the benefits of your weight and aerobic training. So if you are just eating a bowl of oatmeal, you must include a protein source along with that. Here are some examples of protein sources you can have for breakfast.

Example protein sources for breakfast:

- Egg Whites
- Egg Beaters
- Protein Powders (whey, egg, milk, soy)
- Meal Replacement Powders (Optimum Nutrition, Labrada, Met-Rx, Champion Nutrition, etc.)
- Cottage Cheese
- Meat such as, lean cuts of sausage, steak or bacon (if you can handle it in the morning)

Again**, including a protein source will bring you into positive nitrogen balance, increase the metabolism through the digestion of the protein itself, and increase fat mobilization for fuel.** Now that we have the protein source problem solved, what about the complex carbohydrates? Try to stay away from highly processed, sugar loaded cereals. Your best option is to stick with the more natural high-fiber sources such as oatmeal, shredded wheat, fiber cereals etc. These complex carbohydrate sources contain high amounts of vitamins and minerals, and are loaded with fiber.

We need to **consume a minimum of 40 grams of fiber a day**, so you definitely want to include a good amount in your breakfast. Fiber will also slow down the absorption of carbohydrates yielding a steadier supply of energy and a more stable blood sugar level in the body.

Doctor's Prescription:
Fiber is your secret weapon for optimum health. Get a steady supply and it will help you in all areas of health and well-being. Also, if I want a change of pace for breakfast I will eat a bowl of Fiber One cereal along with some protein of some kind.

To put it all together I will use what I had for breakfast as an example. After my 30 minutes of cardiovascular training upon rising I had the following:

- 10 egg whites / 2 yolks
- 2 servings of oatmeal w/ cinnamon
- 12 oz. of water

The meal above contains a balance of good quality protein, high-fiber complex carbohydrates, and a small amount of fat I find I need through out the day. Remember this is just an example; you might need more or less depending on your activity level, and lean muscle mass.

Alcohol and training

I think the most common question that I get is, "will drinking too much hurt my results", and I usually want to yell at the person who asks this question, because they already know the answer. OF COURSE! Honestly, anything in excess is not good.

If you drink moderately, no more than 2-3 drinks per week, you should be OK, but **if you are a heavy drinker, you will never improve your physique.** Understand that alcohol is poisonous to the body and you liver works extra hard to remove it. Your liver would be better served by working on your diet and glycogen levels instead.

Prolonged usage at high doses will:

- reduce your strength - you won't be able to lift enough weight to stimulate muscle growth
- reduce your endurance
- decrease your recovery capabilities - it will take you longer to recuperate and you will be much more sore after workouts
- decrease your aerobic capacity
- reduce your ability to metabolize fat - you will become a fat "storer" instead of a fat "burner"
- interfere with muscle growth
- acts as a diuretic, which can rebound and lead to elevated water retention

Remember, **alcohol** is a totally nutrition less carbohydrate. Even though it's a carb, **it has 7 calories per gram instead of the normal 4.** Like most carbs, it causes the release of insulin, which will cause the storage of your alcohol calories as fat. The constant insulin release will also make it very difficult to lose fat since your body has ample glycogen from the alcohol.

The following table has some useful info on popular beers. So if you go out for a couple of beers you can make an educated decision on which beer is the least damaging to your diet. The figures are for a 12 ounce can or bottle of beer. FYI, Michelob Ultra and Aspen Edge (Coors) are labeled low-carb beers.

Beer data

Brand name	Calories	Carbs (g)	Alcohol (%)
Michelob	155	13.3	5.0
Budweiser	145	10.6	5.0
Miller (MGD)	143	13.1	4.7
Coors	142	10.6	2.0
Michelob Light	134	11.7	4.3
Bud Light	110	6.6	4.2
Coors Light	102	5.0	4.2
Miller Lite	96	3.2	4.2
Michelob Ultra	95	2.6	4.2
Aspen Edge	94	2.6	4.1

Training +nutrition = mass, a sample diet

How do you get the best gains? By training hard and strict - of course. And when you've left the gym the REAL bodybuilding process begins, when you feed your body what it needs to reconstruct and overcompensate while you're resting at home. Make the best use of your biological clock, giving the body exactly what it needs, WHEN it needs it the most.

Enough babble. You wanted it, so here it is, once and for all - the basic eating schedule for good growth.

Meal #1:

The breakfast should always be big. You've been fasting for 8 hours or more by then, so you better do all you can to get out of the catabolic state that's chewing up your muscles for fuel. Get a good 40 grams of protein and a good part of your daily carbs right there and then. I've found oatmeal porridge and eggs to be close to the ultimate breakfast.

Suggestion:

2 large bowls of oatmeal porridge + lowfat milk

6-12 scrambled egg whites + a few yolks

1 glass of orange juice

Multivitamin/mineral capsule

Meal #2:

Snack time. By now you're probably at work or in school, so we want something convenient to just munch on during a ten-minute break, keeping blood sugar up and muscle recovery going.

Suggestion:

1 lean protein bar

or

1 pure protein drink (for non-hardgainers)

1 banana

or

1 gainer drink (mostly carbs, for hardgainers)

1 banana

Meal #3:

Now you need a good, sturdy lunch to keep you going for the rest of the afternoon. As you're going to train right after work/school, you want to start storing a good supply of carbs for workout-energy. Now we're talking pasta, rice or potatoes.

Suggestion:

1 cup of pasta

8-12 ounces of meat of your choice

Steamed carrots & peas

Or

1 cup of rice

2 skinless chicken breasts

Steamed carrots & peas

Meal #4:

Afternoon snack - and pre-workout meal. We want something light yet carb-dense. This is also a good time to take your creatine, and make sure to drink plenty the hour before workout so that you're well-hydrated before you hit the gym.

Suggestion:

1 carb/protein drink

Handful of nuts or sunflower seeds

Or

1 banana

2 rye-sandwiches with lean turkey and lettuce

Meal #5:

Post-workout meal. Now you've trained, and boy, do you want to force-feed your muscles or what? Now you have the chance to stuff your muscles with glycogen (energy for the next workout) at the same time as getting youself into an anabolic state ASAP. Some scientists even claim that if you time it well (i.e., eat within 30-60 mins after training) you'll even increase the body's natural release of growth hormone during the following night!

Suggestion:

1 Gatorade or similar (for once, sugar is GOOD!)

Rice/Potatoes/Pasta-dish + meat of your choice

1-2 fruits of your choice

Meal #6:

Last meal of the day. Now you're going to bed, so you want to avoid carbs (could make you fat). Protein, on the other hand, will be just what your body need to rebuild itself while you're soundly asleep. Aim for low-calorie, low-carb and high-protein. That spells "pure whey-protein drink." And you can have it right before going to bed.

Suggestion:

1 pure protein drink

There you have it, plain and simple. 6 meals throughout the day. No magic, no bull - just good nutrition. If you want to gain weight, you just make sure to get big serving sizes, and when you want to cut up you decrease it slightly. Look at the packages and make notes in your daily log of the total calories. This will help you to adjust your diet properly when you hit a plateau. Unless you're dieting to lose fat, it's OK to have that bag of nachos or something once a week. Just make sure you get good food the rest of the time, and you'll be right on target while keeping morale up. And remember: Don't go overboard with the protein drinks. Food is the foundation, so only resort to supplements when you don't have time to cook. Exception: Last drink before going to bed.

Understanding food labels

At home, you can eat only what is available. For your weight management program to be successful, you must master the art of low-fat shopping. If what you have in your refrigerator and cupboards is junk food, chances are you'll eat that in place of healthy, low-fat foods that satisfy and provide energy.

Before you head to the store, you should have a clear understanding of how to read labels so you can make the healthiest, wisest choices of foods you will enjoy. The following are key words for properly understanding food product labels:

- Serving size: The amount of food the information refers to.
- Servings per container: The number of servings in the entire product or package.
- Percent daily values: Shows how a food fits into an overall daily diet based on a daily intake of 2,000 calories.
- Calories: The total number of calories in one serving of this food.
- Calories from fat: The total number of calories from fat in one serving of this food.
- Total fat: The weight of fat (in grams) in one serving of this food.
- Saturated fat: The weight of saturated fat (in grams) in one serving of this food.
- Sodium: The weight of sodium (in milligrams) in one serving of this food.
- Protein: The weight of protein (in grams) in one serving of this food.

• Total carbohydrates: The weight of both complex and simple carbohydrates (in grams) in one serving of this food.

• Sugars: The weight of simple carbohydrates (in grams) in one serving of this food; to find out how many complex carbohydrates are in the food simply subtract sugars from total carbohydrates.

After you have a clear understanding of the key label words, there are five other important values you will want to consider before concluding that the food product is a healthy, low-fat food.

1. Check the list of ingredients

Ingredients are listed in descending order according to their quantity in that food. The first three or four ingredients listed usually make up most of the product. Keep in mind, however, that fat and sugar come in many different forms, even if they are not one of the first three ingredients, the food can still be very high in fat and/or sugar. Other "names" of fat include hydrogenated vegetable shortening, butter, margarine, oil (coconut, safflower, palm, etc.), lecithin, lard, and cream solids.

Other names of sugars include fructose, honey, corn sweeteners, molasses, maltose, corn syrup, fructose, galactose, glucose, and dextrose. If only one of these names appears among the first few ingredients on the label, or if several of them are listed throughout the label, this food is likely to be high in fat or sugar.

2. Pay attention to total fat and saturated fat

When checking the label of a food, always check the line that reads "total fat." Most experts believe you should get no more than 25 percent of total daily calories from fat. For someone who weighs 160 pounds, that would be about 72 grams a day. So before purchasing any food, check the total fat to see if that product fits into your eating plan.

Right below the "total fat" line is "saturated fat." Again, you want this number to be very low, since this type of fat is linked to obesity and heart disease. **No more than 10 percent of your calories should come from saturated fats.** For the average person, this is between 7-10 grams a day.

The Doctor Says:
In the near future be on the lookout for trans fats. FDA labeling will require the information to be on labels in the next couple of years. The concern is there is growing evidence that trans fats are the worst fats of all. I'll keep you posted as more research becomes available.

---

3. Figure out the percentage of calories from fat

In addition to listing the ingredients, labels give you the information you need to determine the percentage of calories from fat in a specific food product. Knowing this is actually far more important than simply knowing the number of grams of fat in the food product. Just as you want less than 25 percent of your total daily calories to be from fat, you also want to try to eat foods that get less than 25 percent of their total calories from fat. Because a food product has a low number of fat grams, it is not necessarily a low-fat, healthy food.

Take, for example, a reduced-fat whipping cream. Many people assume that since this product only has 1.5 grams of fat per serving that it is a healthy dessert topping (often justifying double or triple the amount on their dessert). However, this product contains actually 45 percent fat. On the other hand, a common nutrition bar has 5 grams of fat per serving. Many dieters would not touch this product for fear of so much fat, when, in actuality, this product contains only 12 percent fat.

How can a food that only has 1.5 grams of fat per serving have a higher percentage of fat calories than a product that contains 5 grams of fat? It is quite simple: The whipped topping only contains 30 calories per serving whereas the nutrition bar contains 380. The nutrition bar is packed with protein and carbohydrates, giving the product a lot more nutritious food value and more calories. Since the whipped topping only contains 30 calories, it has very little nutritional value and quite a bit of fat relative to the total volume of food and calories. When checking labels, be sure to figure out the percentage of fat calories in addition to the number of fat grams.

To determine the percentage of calories from fat of a food product, look for two important numbers: calories per serving and total grams of fat per serving. Since you want to know what percentage of the total calories are fat calories, you must first convert the grams of fat into calories. Remember, there are 9 calories per gram of fat.

To calculate the fat percentage of the food:

a) Multiply the number of grams of fat by the number 9.

b) Divide this number by the total calories per serving.

c) The result is the percentage of fat calories (should be less than 25).

Food label terms, what they really mean

The FDA has created rules regarding the use of certain terms on food labels. To understand what the food actually contains, you must know what these terms mean.

Calorie Terms

- **"Low Calorie"** = Contains no more than 40 calories per serving.
- **"Reduced Calorie"** = Contains 25% fewer calories per serving than regular product
- **"Calorie-Free"** = Contains less than 5 calories per serving

Sodium Terms

- **"Low Sodium"** = Containing 140mg of sodium or less per serving.
- **"Very Low Sodium"** = Containing 35mg of sodium or less per serving.

Fat Terms (non-meat)

- **"Fat-Free"** = Contains no more than 0.5g of fat per serving.

- **"Low Cholesterol"** = Contains no more than 20g of cholesterol and less than 2g of saturated fat per serving.
- **"Low Fat"** = Contains no more than 3g of fat per serving

Fat Terms (meat products)

- **"Lean"** = Contains no more than 10g of fat, no more than 4.5g of which is saturated fat, also contains less than 95mg of cholesterol per serving
- **"Extra Lean"** = Contains no more than 5g of fat, no more than 2g of which is saturated fat, also contains less than 95mg of cholesterol per serving

Other Terms

- **"Free", "No", "Zero"** = Containing no amount, or a trivial amount
- **"Sugar-Free"** = Containing less than 0.5g per serving
- **"Good Source"** = Provides 10%-19% of Daily Value per serving

"Light" = Can mean one of three things:

a) provides 1/3 fewer calories or 1/2 the amount of fat as the regular product per serving

b) if it's a "low fat", "low-calorie" food, it can be called "light" if it provides 1/2 the normal fat present

c) can be referring to the actual color of the food itself

10 biggest nutritional mistakes

Larry Scott, the first Mr. Olympia, remarked in 1965 'Bodybuilding is 90% nutrition.' Shawn Ray in 1993 echoed the sentiment: 'The weights, the gym, the training, I can do that part in my sleep; it's fun and relatively easy. It's the other stuff, the dieting and supplementing, that demands the discipline.' If success is any measure, Shawn knoweth that of which he speaketh. Top professional bodybuilders weight, measure, quantify and chart every bite they put into their mouths.

Does the grass roots trainer need to go to that level of dedication and exactitude? To maximize gains, yes. Perhaps not to the degree the elite go to, but nutrition is a key ingredient in bodybuilding success. So take a hint. Without a scientific nutrition program, bodybuilding devolves into plan weight training, which is a hell of a lot further down athletic evolution. As Robby Robinson once observed 'Nutrition is everything'.

Taoist monks in search of spiritual enlightenment have a method for obtaining nirvana called, the Negative Way. In the system of Wu Wei, adherents obtain enlightenment through negation. Rather than try to define the enlightened truth, they identify all that is false. After doing so, they are left with that which is true. Hidden within the science that encapsulates modern bodybuilding nutrition, we have the equivalent of Wu Wei. We can acquire nutritional truth through the identification of that which is false. Identifying the false sheds light on its opposite, the truth. Here are the top 10 false moves of bodybuilding nutrition and their implied opposites.

1. Eating too much

We all know the biology. Excess calories are stored as body fat. For overeating to be at the top of the nutritional false move list is no mistake. Building muscle is the number one goal of bodybuilding and body fat is the bodybuilder's number one enemy. What's the sense of working an impressive set of muscles requiring much blood, sweat and tears, if a layer of lard obscures it? May I suggest the obvious? If you are overweight, eat less. The simple act on consuming less food will cause you to lose weight.

Be aware, however, that if you eat less but retain your current food profile, you will just construct a miniature version of your old self. Less of the same will shrink you, but your proportion of muscle to body fat will stay the same. The end result? You look like your old self, just pounds lighter. Truly sensational physical transformation lies in losing body fat while maintaining muscle. To achieve true nutritional nirvana, building muscle while simultaneously losing body fat, we need to practice nutrient based dieting.

To lose fat and retain muscle, besides doing aerobic exercise, you need to eat precise amounts of protein, carbohydrates and fat. You need to become nutrient conscious. Read the labels on the food you eat. What is the consensus on achieving metabolic nirvana? To hang on to muscle, you need protein and lots of it. To maintain energy and fuel growth you need quality cards. To shed the fat blanket and keep the muscle, to effect the physical transformation you seek, you need lots of quality nutrients, but not in excess. You tread the razor's edge between enough and too much. Everyone is different. Experiment and monitor.

2. Eating too little

Under eating is as bad as overeating. Physiologically, it's impossible to build muscle if your diet lacks proper nutrients. Ample amounts of protein, carbohydrates, and yes, even fat are necessary to build muscle. The trick is balance; you need enough high quality food to grow muscle. Yet even the finest muscle fuel will be stored as fat if taken in excess. One key strategy is to confine your eating to 'clean fuel', nutritionally dense foods with little or no fat and sugar. And you need to eat plenty of them. A serious weight trainer who additionally performs regular cardiovascular work will need to the extra nutrients to cope with the additional metabolic demands.

3. Insufficient protein

The fact remains: Protein is the single most important nutrient for muscle regeneration and building. The trick is to use only lean protein. Protein and fat usually coexist in food sources.

Meat, fish, fowl, dairy, these primary sources all can have much fat content. In the old days, we did not worry about such inconveniences. As a result, heavy protein consumers developed nasty clogged arteries and astronomical cholesterol rates. The fault wasn't in the protein, but the fat attached to the protein.

Nowadays, we hardcore weight trainers confine our protein to nonfat or low fat sources. Skim milk, egg whites, fish, skinless fowl, flank steak, and of course that staple of weight training, protein powder. These foods represent powerful, clean protein sources. Start by ingesting 1 - 1.5 grams of protein per pound of bodyweight per day. To stay anabolic, divide the total intake into 4-8 equal portions and eat these low fat protein sources at regular intervals throughout the day.

4. Failing to cook for yourself

Meal preparation is a critical skill. To be truly successful as a bodybuilder, you should be able to prepare your own food. Nutritionally sound foods eaten throughout the day are necessary to obtain anabolism. Most male bodybuilders (and more than a few female ones) do not cook. Big mistake. Why depend on mom, your spouse, restaurants or fast food joints for the endless succession of small, nutritious feedings required to mount a serious bodybuilder effort?

Not only do you have to come to grips with cooking, but also you have to develop a wide and inventive repertoire of dishes and meals. Otherwise you are locked into the equivalent of prison chow. Jailhouse cuisine is bland, unimaginative, and tasteless. Kind of like the clean foods we bodybuilders choose to contend with day in, day out.

You need a lot of imagination to deal with clean food. Tuna and egg white need not be dull. How do the ignorant become enlightened? Comb the magazines. Read low fat cookbooks. Assemble your ingredients, set aside some time and have at it. Plus, you'll impress the heck out of your mom when you serve her a low fat gourmet feast some fine Sunday.

5. Not keeping a nutrition log

As cumbersome as it might sound, the muscle elite keep daily records of what they consume and when they consume it. They write it all down in a log. This allows them to keep a running tally of their nutritional progress. They establish a long-term game plan and keep daily tabs on food and supplement consumption. Tracking results, identifying trends, finding what works, discarding what doesn't, and a log becomes your nutritional report card. You can make truly accurate assessments and implement intelligent corrective action when you base your adjustments on factual data and objective analysis. Otherwise it degenerates into wishful thinking and self-delusion.

So begin by assembling data. The truly complete nutritional log lists date, time, food type, and carb, fat, sugar, sodium, protein and caloric content. Body stats are notated along with short descriptive phrases on the athlete's general condition. Drawn up in column format, the comprehensive notation of a meal takes about two minutes. And you'll find that the purchases of a food nutritional value book (available at any bookstore) will be of a great help. Did I hear you say what a hassle? It could be worse. Thomas Jefferson wrote down every financial transaction he made in his adult life and he lived to be 83.

6. Too much fat & sugar

The twin demons of nutrition. Fat is calorically the densest of all nutrients, with nine calories per gram. Fat is hard to digest and is the body's preferred storage material. Though a certain amount of fat is needed for brain and other bodily functions, the little that's required is easily acquired through regular low fat eating.

Excess sugar is easily converted to fat once in the body. Buyers beware: A food may be advertised as low fat and still be loaded with sugar. Taken in excess, this sugar can be quickly converted to fat. Quite a few a few of the sports drinks and nutritional sports bars are loaded with sugar. Limit fat intake to roughly 15% of your total caloric consumption.

7. Not drinking enough water

As we know, the body is 67% water, and we should drink lots of water throughout the day. Water courses throughout the body's plumbing; downing copious amounts throughout the day keeps the pipes clean as chrome. So flush the system continually and regularly, regenerating muscle cells through water replenishment. Drink 10 eight-ounce glasses of water a day.

8. Lacking positive nitrogen balance

Positive nitrogen balance is the physiological state in which muscular growth is possible. How to achieve it? Take in a fresh supply of muscle building nutrients every 2-3 hours. The human body works most efficiently when given small feedings at regular intervals throughout the day. These evenly spaced feedings should be composed of high quality protein and carbohydrates.

How can you eat every 2-3 hours when faced with the rigors of a job, family and real world responsibilities? A nutritious sports bar and a glass of skim milk can supply 50 grams of protein and 50-100 grams of carbohydrates. How long does it take to eat a sandwich? Or drink a protein shake? How about a piece of fruit and a chicken breast? You get the idea. This ties into food preparation; pack clean food snacks and graze throughout the day. When an athlete is in positive nitrogen balance, the body is ready, willing and able to grow.

9. Lacking food balance in meals

Imbalance is rampant in this off kilter world. Food consumption is no exception. Balanced eating as defined by some nutritionists is not quite the same as balanced eating as defined by the muscle elite. The optimal feeding, according to the elite, is a skillful blending of lean protein, starchy and fibrous carbohydrates, minuscule amounts of fat and no sugar. The proportional divisions vary depending upon individual characteristics. Some folks are carb sensitive and need to keep starchy carbs to a minimum, otherwise they blow up like cartoon characters who've swallowed an air hose. Others thrive on a diet heavy on potatoes and rice with no ill effects.

How you metabolize food is as individual as your hair color or height. You need to determine how foods affect you. Rule of thumb for proportional balance: 50% calories from carbs, 35% from protein and 15% from fat. This is a good starting point, and careful monitoring once on this 50-35-15 regimen will dictate any necessary adjustments.

The goal is building muscle and reducing body fat. How do you achieve a real world balance with traveling around with a scale, calorie book, and calculator? At each meal, fill 50% of your plate with carbohydrates. Half of these should be dense, starchy carbs (rice, potatoes) and half should be fibrous carbs (broccoli, green beans, lettuce, etc.). The other half of the dinner plate should consist of lean protein (skinless chicken, turkey, fish, etc.). Don't worry about the 15% fat... it's there!

10. Ignoring supplementation

We all have little holes and shortcomings in our diets, and supplements help us round them out. All elite athletes use supplements. The expense, hassle and confusion of diet supplementing scares off some trainers. Big mistake. State with a prepackaged multipack. In addition, a quality protein powder, a high-grade carbohydrate powder, and a big supply if beef liver tabs will do wonders for your recuperation, training, and physique.

Ten tips for eating well despite your busy schedule

The biggest obstacle you may face when trying to implement a bodybuilding nutritional program is to do so despite your busy schedule at work and at play. Oftentimes, it seems that everything else takes priority over eating correctly. In the short run, it's easier to just skip an important meal like breakfast rather than getting yourself out of bed just 10 minutes earlier to eat. It's convenient to stop at Burger King for a Whopper and fries rather than going home, cooking a chicken breast, rice, and vegetables, and cleaning up the mess afterwards.

And you know what? You're right! It is much easier to skip meals or stop for fast food. But, if you want to build a physique that you can be proud of, you must make the decision to eat correctly.

I'll be perfectly honest with you, there are no "secrets." The bottom line is you have to make the commitment to change. Eating right can't be something you "should" do; it has to be something you "must" do if you want to have the body you desire. Everything worth having takes extra effort. Your body is no exception. Let's face it; if it were easy, everybody would have a fantastic physique!

Here are ten tips I've discovered to make the process of eating the way you should despite your busy schedule a little easier:

1. **Organization and advanced planning are essential.** Plan ahead and create diet menus for the entire week, then go to the grocery store and purchase all the food you will need. Don't get caught short of the food you'll need to support your bodybuilding efforts. You'll be less likely to go back to the store in the middle of your busy week.

2. **Choose food containers that will make eating more convenient.** Rubbermaid "Servin' Saver" food containers are ideal for eating on the go. Ziploc plastic bags are very versatile and will keep your food fresh. Smaller ice chests come in a variety of fashionable and convenient sizes that can keep your food cold while you're driving around in your car or sitting at your desk.

3. **Get in the habit of carrying water with you at all times.** More and more people are discovering the benefits of drinking 8 glasses of water a day, and those "spring water" bottles are becoming more and more visible. You won't see me anywhere without my one-gallon plastic jug of water nearby.

4. **Make time to eat smaller meals throughout the day.** If you plan ahead and cook your meals FOR THE ENTIRE DAY the night before or in the morning, you can warm up a container of pre-cooked food in the microwave. In the middle of your busy day, preparing meals will take only a few minutes. When you calculate all the time you'll save each meal, staying on schedule will be a little less overwhelming. As a bodybuilder, you should eat *at least* 5 or 6 times a day. Your body will use food more efficiently eating smaller, more frequent meals instead of eating the traditional three larger meals.

5. **Take advantage of modern food preparation technology.** There are many appliances on the market that make preparing meals a lot easier and faster. Bigger muscles, lower body fat, better health, and greater self-esteem are well worth the investment. People on the go should always have access to a microwave oven. If you don't have an automatic rice cooker, make a point of getting one today. I highly recommend the George Foreman Grill as well.

6. **Although some people believe fresh vegetables are best for you, don't be afraid to take advantage of the convenience of frozen vegetables.** There is only a slight difference in the nutritional values of frozen vegetables versus fresh ones. They are definitely easier to prepare and are relatively inexpensive. Busy people just don't have time to clean and cut fresh vegetables. Instead of excluding these important foods, just take them out of the freezer and put them into your food container before you leave for work. By the time of your mid-morning meal, they should be thawed. If you have access to a microwave, delicious hot veggies will be ready to eat in only a few minutes.

7. **Don't get so overly "scientific" about eating that you never get started on a structured program.** Just make sure you eat all the food you need. Put the entire day's worth of food in one container and eat even amounts throughout the day. Also, don't think you are doing yourself a favor by not eating all the food that you should. Remember, eating a higher amount of calories—without eating in excess—will help build muscle. This will also keep your metabolism raised and thereby help reduce body fat.

8. **Take advantage of convenient "food (or meal) replacements."** Whether it is Ny-Tro Pro 40, MyoPlex, Rx Fuel, Met-Rx, or Mesotech, food replacements are excellent alternatives to regular food. They take the guesswork out of eating properly because they already contain the right proportion of protein, carbohydrates, and fat. This can be especially helpful in sticking to your commitment—even with your busy schedule.

9. **I like pouring my meal replacements into a bowl, mixing them up in a little bit of water,** and mixing the two to create a pudding-like consistency. Not only is the method a lot easier and faster to prepare than making a shake with a blender, I also get the sensation of eating real food. This sensation sure feels good when I'm on a calorie-deprived diet!

10. **At all times, keep a plastic container in your car or at your desk at work** with a few meal replacements, a smaller container of whey protein, a couple of cans of tuna, a smaller bottle of water, a can opener, and some eating utensils. Doing so will make sure that you are NEVER caught short of the food you'll need to support your bodybuilding efforts.

Protein shakes; these have to be your best friend

Protein shakes are an easy way to make sure that your meeting your protein requirements. Protein shakes can be made from protein powders or purchased as prepackaged protein drinks. Each has its advantages and disadvantages. Protein powers are sold at health food stores, supermarkets, and the Internet. There are two types of protein powders:

Total nutrition or complete meal replacement protein

The best meal replacement proteins are derived from a composite of normal milk proteins (casein and whey) and contain at least 30 grams of protein. They also include a complete array of vitamins and minerals, including trace elements. Meal replacement proteins come in different flavors and can be mixed with water or low-fat milk. Many of these products taste pretty good; the only disadvantage is you don't always have a blender around to mix them. There are several brands to choose from. When you shop for one of these products be sure to look for label that says "total nutrition or complete meal replacement protein" on the label.

Pure protein powder

A pure protein powder contains protein and nothing else. **A good protein power provides up to 50 grams of protein per serving.** Pure protein powders are useful because they can be made into high potency protein drinks or used with cooking to enhance the protein content of meals. Pure protein powder is less expensive than the ready to drink replacement protein drinks, but remember it doesn't contain the same full complement of nutrients. **I usually recommend that people drink at least one meal replacement drink daily** to make sure that they're getting all their nutrients. If you choose to drink an additional protein drink, a pure protein power is a more economical alternative. Also, if you're on a low to moderate carb diet you should go for the pure protein powder drinks for all your meal replacement shakes.

What about people who are lactose intolerant? Most adults experience some form of lactose intolerance, ranging from the mild to the severe. The lactose content is so minimal in many brands of protein powder that it usually does not cause problems. If you know you are lactose intolerant, try drinking a small amount of the shake and see if it causes any adverse reaction. In all likelihood you'll not have any problems. Don't mix your shakes with milk. Use water. You can also try taking a lactate pill before drinking your shake. However, if you're one of those people who cannot tolerate even the tiniest amount of lactose, I recommended you avoid these products and get your protein from food.

Let's also talk about protein bars

Protein bars (also called food bars, meal replacement bars, and energy bars) can be a convenient and portable ways to augment your protein intake on the run. But be careful: some protein bars are little more than candy bars in disguise! To make sure that you are getting a high-quality protein bar, read the label. **A high-quality protein bar should be at least 30 to 50 percent protein by weight.** For example if the protein bar weighs 100 grams, it should contain at least 30 to 50 grams of protein.

Doctor's Prescription:
So far to date, I have tried dozens of protein bars and for the most part they are tasteless bricks. However they have come a long way in the last few years. Labrada Nutrition probably has the best tasting bar with a decent nutritional profile that I have tried.

Also, be aware of added sugar. Shockingly, the case in many bars, sugar is the first, second, or third and ingredient listed on the label. These bars contain a lot more sugar than protein! Also, many protein bars contain high amounts of high fructose corn sugar. **I don't recommend any protein bar in which sugar or high fructose corn syrup is listed as one of the three top ingredients.** For the same reasons mentioned above, I would avoid protein bars in which soy is a primary source of protein.

Whey protein

From an athlete's point of view, whey proteins are highly digestible and have a better amino acid profile even than egg whites. Let me say that again: **whey protein has the highest biological value of any protein.**

It's absorbed, utilized and retained better. This higher biological value makes whey more tissue sparing, making it a benefit to people as they diet, age, overtrain or have illnesses or disease. Whey is high in the BCAA's, which are the aminos most oxidized during exercise and may decrease muscle soreness thru its quadra-peptides, which have pain killing qualities. It assists in recovery from athletic activity and may contribute to bone cell growth, potentially strengthening all the bones in the aging human body.

Aside from the tissue repair qualities found in other proteins, **whey protein is an immune system enhancer;** it boosts the body's ability to fight infection and in some studies has been shown to even inhibit the growth of cancer cells. Intense training lowers immune system response, whey boosts immune response.

Whey assists in building up the body's own antioxidants by raising the levels of glutathione, an essential water-soluble antioxidant that protects the cells and neutralizes toxins. It's a first line immune system defense; it inhibits the growth of iron-dependent bacteria, scavenges free iron, can block the growth of pathogenic bacteria and yeast, can stimulate the beneficial intestinal micro flora and has antibacterial properties.

Sub-fractions of whey concentrate stimulate insulin-like growth factor (IGF-1) production (closely tied to growth hormone), which increases muscle and tendon strength and contributes to injury repair. Casein and colostrum are apparently factors in the IGF stimulation in the body as well, but the studies are sketchy. The added casein inhibits whole-body protein breakdown, it's anti-catabolic, which whey protein is not. Whey also stimulates the release of cholecystokinin (CCK), which decreases the appetite.

Whey isolates, by the way, do not produce these benefits. The acid process required to make the isolate does increase the protein content over whey concentrate, but destroys the sub-fractions (the lactoferrins, beta-lactoglobulins, immuno-globulins, etc.), which are some of the more potent immune system and antioxidant features of whey proteins. As we age, these sub-fractions become more important. My understanding is that the whey isolate process is more expensive, so in that the labels may be true.

On the other hand, protein labels that guarantee a certain percentage of these sub-fractions are probably not accurate as these sub-fractions are dependent upon uncontrollable circumstances such as feed, rainfall, breed of cow, age of cow, etc. So if your protein makes precise percentage claims it may be bogus.

30 grams of whey protein a day can do all this. Since I started this research, I went from occasional protein drinks when I couldn't get food to a protein drink a day as my most important meal, usually 2 protein drinks or more per day.

Creatine: More than a sports nutrition supplement

Although creatine offers an array of benefits, most people think of it simply as a supplement that bodybuilders and other athletes use to gain strength and muscle mass. Nothing could be further from the truth.

A substantial body of research has found that creatine may have a wide variety of uses. In fact, creatine is being studied as a supplement that may help with diseases affecting the neuromuscular system, such as muscular dystrophy (MD). Recent studies suggest creatine may have therapeutic applications in aging populations for wasting syndromes, muscle atrophy, fatigue, gyrate atrophy, Parkinson's disease, Huntington's disease and other brain pathologies. Several studies have shown creatine can reduce cholesterol by up to 15% and it has been used to correct certain inborn errors of metabolism, such as in people born without the enzymes responsible for making creatine. Some studies have found that creatine may increase growth hormone production.

What is creatine?

Creatine is formed in the human body from the amino acids methionine, glycine and arginine. **The average person's body contains approximately 120 grams of creatine stored as creatine phosphate. Certain foods such as beef, herring and salmon, are fairly high in creatine.** However, a person would have to eat pounds of these foods daily to equal what can be obtained in one teaspoon of powdered creatine.

Creatine is directly related to adenosine triphosphate (ATP). ATP is formed in the powerhouses of the cell, the mitochondria. ATP is often referred to as the "universal energy molecule" used by every cell in our bodies. An increase in oxidative stress coupled with a cell's inability to produce essential energy molecules such as ATP, is a hallmark of the aging cell and is found in many disease states. Key factors in maintaining health are the ability to: (a) prevent mitochondrial damage to DNA caused by reactive oxygen species (ROS) and (b) prevent the decline in ATP synthesis, which reduces whole body ATP levels. It would appear that maintaining antioxidant status (in particular intra-cellular glutathione) and ATP levels are essential in fighting the aging process.

It is interesting to note that many of the most promising anti-aging nutrients such as CoQ10, NAD, acetyl-l-carnitine and lipoic acid are all taken to maintain the ability of the mitochondria to produce high energy compounds such as ATP and reduce oxidative stress. The ability of a cell to do work is directly related to its ATP status and the health of the mitochondria. Heart tissue, neurons in the brain and other highly active tissues are very sensitive to this system. Even small changes in ATP can have profound effects on the tissues' ability to function properly. Of all the nutritional supplements available to us currently, creatine appears to be the most effective for maintaining or raising ATP levels.

How does creatine work?

In a nutshell, creatine works to help generate energy. When ATP loses a phosphate molecule and becomes adenosine diphosphate (ADP), it must be converted back to ATP to produce energy. Creatine is stored in the human body as creatine phosphate (CP) also called phosphocreatine. When ATP is depleted, CP can recharge it. That is, CP donates a phosphate molecule to the ADP, making it ATP again. An increased pool of CP means faster and greater recharging of ATP, which means more work can be performed. This is why creatine has been so successful for athletes. For short-duration explosive sports, such as sprinting, weight lifting and other anaerobic endeavors, ATP is the energy system used.

The Doctor Says:
I know that my creatine explanation may sound overly scientific but it is important for you to understand how it works. Since it is such a popular supplement today, it will benefit you to know the topic in detail.

To date, **research has shown that ingesting creatine can increase the total body pool of CP,** which leads to greater generation of energy for anaerobic forms of exercise, such as weight training and sprinting. **Other effects of creatine may be increases in protein synthesis and increased cell hydration.**

Creatine has had spotty results in affecting performance in endurance sports such as swimming, rowing and long distance running, with some studies showing no positive effects on performance in endurance athletes. Whether or not the failure of creatine to improve performance in endurance athletes was due to the nature of the sport or the design of the studies is still being debated.

Creatine can be found in the form of creatine monohydrate, creatine citrate, creatine phosphate, creatine-magnesium chelate and even liquid versions. However, the vast majority of research to date showing creatine to have positive effects on pathologies, muscle mass and performance used the monohydrate form. **Creatine monohydrate is over 90% absorbable.**

How to get the best gains from creatine

Creatine is probably the most talked about supplement on the market. It is one of the few supplements that can produce noticeable gains in lean mass, strength, and energy in a very short time. Most people find that within a week of taking creatine their muscles become fuller and they get better pumps when working out.

Creatine is a natural substance produced in our bodies to supply energy. Creatine is formed from the amino acids arginine, methionine, and glycine. Creatine is used to produce chemical energy called adenosine triphosphate (ATP). The average person produces approximately 2 grams of creatine per day. This is enough to maintain a creatine balance.

Creatine supplementation raises blood creatinine, but it is not toxic or harmful in healthy individuals. Creatine is found in the foods that we eat especially protein foods such as meats and fish. Vegetarians usually have a very low intake of creatine.

Muscles consist of approximately 75% water. Creatine helps to draw water into the muscle cells producing what is called cell-volumization. This makes the muscles feel full and pumped. **Studies show that when a muscle cell is volumized it helps to stimulate protein synthesis and minimize protein breakdown.**

Twelve test subjects performed 5 bouts of 30 voluntary knee extensions with 1 minute recovery periods between each bout. Subjects were tested for peak muscle torque production before and after treatment with either placebo or creatine. The treatment period lasted 5 days and consisted of a placebo 4 times a day or 5g of creatine 4 times a day plus 1g of glucose a day. Subjects who were administered the placebo demonstrated no difference in performance. In the creatine group, however, peak muscle torque production increased in all subjects during the final 10 contractions of exercise in bout 1, throughout the entirety of exercise in bouts 2, 3, and 4, and during contractions 11-20 of bout 5 after supplementation. Researchers concluded that creatine supplementation increased the level of peak torque production during repeated bouts of maximal voluntary muscle contractions.

In a similar study, researchers divided sixteen test subjects into two groups receiving either 20g per day creatine monohydrate, or placebo (glucose), for a six-day treatment period. Before and after the treatment period, subjects performed high-intensity exercise consisting of 10 six-second bouts on a cycle ergometer with a 30 second recovery period in between attempting to maintain a pedaling frequency of 140 revolutions per minute. There was no difference in exercise output between the two groups before the treatment period.

After treatment, however, the group supplementing with creatine monohydrate displayed an easier time maintaining the target speed towards the end of each exercise bout than the placebo group. One of the best ways to take creatine is to mix a level teaspoonful of creatine (approx. 5 grams) with a glass of Kool-Aid or some other high sugar drink. The reason for the high sugar is to cause your body to release insulin; this will allow your muscles to absorb the creatine much better. There have been several studies done which prove that taking creatine with insulin releasing carbohydrates (sugars) increases the uptake of creatine by the muscle cells.

Doctor's Prescription:
I have mentioned a couple of the scientific studies on creatine here but you should go to the library and do your own research on journal articles and other publications so you have a better understanding of what is true and what is not true when you read product labels.

I have experimented with several different methods of using creatine and I find that the best way to use it is simply have 4-5 grams of creatine in the morning mixed in a protein shake. And take another 4-5 grams of creatine after your workouts. When you take creatine after your workouts make sure you add it to a high sugar drink as I mentioned before to get the extra insulin spike. The metabolic environment created by a hard workout will allow your muscles to absorb the creatine really well. On the days that you do not workout, just take 4-5 grams once a day mixed in a protein shake.

Your body's natural creatine production will eventually stop if you don't take some time off from creatine supplementation. Because of this you will get better results by cycling on and off creatine, then if you just took it all of the time. I recommend that you use it for a couple of months and then take one month off before using it again.

Creatine conclusion

Creatine is quickly becoming one of the best researched and promising supplements for a wide range of diseases. It may have additional uses for pathologies where a lack of high-energy compounds and general muscle weakness exist, such as fibromyalgia. People with fibromyalgia have lower levels of creatine phosphate and ATP levels compared to controls. Some studies also suggest it helps with the strength and endurance of healthy but aging people as well. Though additional research is needed, **there is a substantial body of research showing creatine is an effective and safe supplement for a wide range of pathologies and may be the next big find in anti-aging nutrients.**

Although the doses used in some studies were quite high, recent studies suggest lower doses are just as effective for increasing the overall creatine phosphate pool in the body. Two to three grams per day appears adequate for healthy people to increase their tissue levels of creatine phosphate. People with the aforementioned pathologies or bodybuilders may benefit from higher intakes, in the 5-to-10 grams per day range.

Glutamine, the best amino acid

When you look at any bodybuilding or fitness magazine you see dozens of ads for supplements that all promise to give you huge gains in muscle and a reduction in bodyfat. Very few people can afford to take them all. And if you did you would spend all day popping pills and forcing down powders, drinks, etc. However, one supplement that you should consider taking is glutamine.

Glutamine is the most abundant amino acid in the body. It constitutes more than 50% of the amino acids found in muscle cells. Glutamine is a non-essential amino acid. Now that term can be a bit confusing. Non-essential simply means that you don't have to get your glutamine from outside sources. It is so important to bodily functions that the body actually produces glutamine.

But your body can only produce a certain amount of glutamine. When you put stress on your body (i.e. exercise) the demand for glutamine increases and very often the body can't produce enough. Our bodies use a lot of glutamine every single day. It is required to maintain the proper function of your immune system, brain, kidneys, pancreas, gall bladder, liver, etc. This places a very high demand on your body's resources.

The brain, organs, immune system, etc. receive high priority for glutamine. Any glutamine that is not used for the essential bodily functions is used to help build and repair muscle tissue. If you don't provide extra glutamine you could easily deplete your body's resources before your muscles receive all the glutamine that they need.

Building muscle is not the body's top priority. **If the body needs extra glutamine for the essential bodily functions it will break down muscle tissue to get the extra glutamine.** This is something that we want to prevent from happening.

Doctor's Prescription:
Add glutamine to your supplementation diet, it is one of the best supplements you can buy. Creatine, glutamine and a multivitamin are the top 3 supplements you will ever use.

This is where supplementation comes in. Studies have shown that supplementing glutamine can prevent muscle wasting; it produces a potent anti-catabolic effect. So what is the best way to supplement glutamine? Consuming an **additional 10 grams of glutamine** along with a high protein diet should do the trick for most bodybuilding and fitness enthusiasts.

I recommend using pure glutamine powder and take 5 grams of glutamine 2 times per day, after a workout and before bed. It is best to take a couple of small servings of glutamine throughout the day because the body can only utilize a small amount of glutamine at one time. You can mix glutamine with either a glass of water, juice, protein drink, etc.

When I started supplementing with glutamine I noticed the results within a week of taking it. I felt better physically and I had more energy in the gym. **I also noticed a reduction in muscle soreness and fatigue.** I highly recommend that you give it a try.

Growth hormone

What is it and where does it come from?

Growth Hormone, a polypeptide hormone secreted by the anterior pituitary gland that regulates tissue growth, cellular repair, energy levels, fat loss, and muscle growth. This is the latest advance in bodybuilding supplementation!

Growth Hormone (GH) is the master hormone, because the master gland; the anterior pituitary gland, releases it. While GH is not necessary or critical to one's survival, it seems to play an important evolutionary role in human development. During puberty, GH levels dictate a person's height and bone size. After puberty, GH continues to regulate the body's metabolism.

What does it do and how can it help a bodybuilder?

Human Growth Hormone levels decline after age 30 give or take a year. These HGH levels, along with the related IGF-1 amounts, must be elevated in order to maximize muscular size and growth. **Human Growth Hormone levels are associated with decreased fat, increased muscle mass, high energy, and increased sex drive.** It is HGH that has been found in studies to facilitate the metabolism of fats in the body. HGH is also known for its powerful muscle-building effects. Increasing HGH is definitely a good thing, especially for bodybuilders. HGH tends to decrease naturally with age, so the older you get, the harder it is to lose fat.

Metabolically speaking, GH is responsible for the regulation of insulin (glucose metabolism), protein synthesis, transportation of amino acids across cell membranes, growth factor-1 (a metabolic liver hormone) and IGF-2, osteablast production (bone mass) and fat metabolism. GH also has a profound effect on the immune system.

During fetal brain development, GH works closely to stimulate IGF-2 production; known to be one of the primary hormones responsible for cognitive development and IQ in children. IGF-2 is the growth factor, which stimulates brain cell growth and development.

Between the ages of 30 and 35, GH production begins a steady decline, and research associates this correspondence with the phenomena we call aging. Somatopause (Soma = GH) is the term used to describe this condition. The human brain shrinks in size by as much as 25% by the time we die, as do other vital organs. Much of this is due to the dramatic drop in the production of somatomedins (growth factors) with age, which in turn are regulated by GH. Within the psychological domain, when GH levels drop, mood levels become less stable and the feelings of youthful resilience (the ability to "bounce back") diminishes.

GH is one of the most extensively researched hormones in the body. **Anti-aging specialists focus on its ability to regenerate kidney, lung, heart, and liver tissue.** The majority of GH research has focused on its clinical application at injectable dosage levels (from 1 to 2 I.U.s). However, research is now surfacing regarding the effects of micro-dilution supplementation on quality of life.

Until 1996, GH was cost-prohibitive for the average American, available in injectable form only. Fortunately, in 1996, due to the development of advanced delivery systems, Americans were presented with other viable options, oral spray micro-dilution supplementation, and cap/tab supplementation.

Human Growth Hormone (HGH) has been extensively studied both clinically and theoretically for many decades. **GH has been referred to as the "Fountain of Youth".** It has astounded the medical community with its numerous positive physiological effects on degenerative conditions related to both aging and disease. The reported higher energy levels, enhanced libido and sexual performance, re-growth of internal organs that shrink with age, and greater cardiac output. In addition, superior immune function, better kidney function, lowering of blood pressure, and improved cholesterol profile (higher HDL and lower LDL) has been documented. Younger, thicker skin with tightening and lessening of wrinkles, hair growth, sharper vision, mood elevation/relief from depression, increased memory retention, improved sleep, decreased recovery time from exercise, muscle strain/injury, and regeneration of tissues in degenerative diseases have also been noted.

HGH supplementation works on the hypothalmic-pituitary axis and follows the natural sequence of GH production by stimulating the hypothalamus to produce GHRH, which in turn stimulates the anterior pituitary to release Somatotropin. Revostatin is a Somatostatin suppressant. Somatostatin is the antagonistic hormone that blocks growth hormone production when blood levels of Somatotropin and IGF-1 rise.

For reversal of the aging process as an aid to both male and female athletes seeking to safely increase their natural GH production. HGH should not be administered to persons who have not completed their bone growth without first consulting a health care professional familiar with HGH therapy. In general, **HGH supplementation is reserved for individuals over age 20.**

The Doctor Says:
Human Growth Hormone is a master hormone because it influences so many different sub-systems within the body. It will help you build muscle, lose fat and look / feel younger. With scientific advancements this supplement will become more affordable in the near future.

No adverse side effects have been reported when used as directed. Follow the directions and recommendations per individual supplement. Recent studies have shown that the effervescent HGH products are the best. The tablets/capsules are second best, and the spray products are last. Of course, there are different opinions on this so if something has been working for you, stick with it.

All about green tea

I have been a green tea fanatic long before the green tea craze hit the supplement market. Now every weight loss product on the market has stuck some green tea extract on their ingredient list. I believe you can get some benefit from supplementing this way but you're not using the plants full potential.

Green Tea Contains The Following:

Tannins - A group of simple and complex phenol, polyphenol, and flavonoid compounds. Produced by plants, all of the tannins are relatively resistant to digestion or fermentation. All tannins act as astringents, shrinking tissues and contracting structural proteins in the skin and mucosa.

Having a cup of green tea after a meal can aid in digestion. Green tea has been used for thousand of years in Asia as a digestive agent.

Catechins - Catechins are a category of polyphenols. In green tea, catechins are present in significant quantities, more specifically, epicatechin (EC), epigallocatechin (EGC), epicatechin gallate (ECG) and epigallocatechin gallate (EGCG). EGCG makes up about 10-50% of the total catechin content and appears to be the most powerful of the catechins with antioxidant activity about 25-100 times more potent than vitamins C and E. A cup of green tea may provide 10-40mg of polyphenols and has antioxidant activity greater than a serving of broccoli, spinach, carrots or strawberries.

All this adds up to having a powerful anti-oxidant coursing through your system after a heavy workout is just what you need to curb free radical damage.

Flavonoids - Flavonoids are plant pigments, and are the brightly colored chemical constituents found in most fresh fruits and vegetables. They may aid in protecting against infection. Deficiency can result in a tendency to bruise easily.

Obviously your workouts will suffer if you are sick. Because your muscles will get sore easier and take longer to heal.

Theanine - An amino acid that produces tranquilizing effects in the brain. Theanine is a unique amino acid found in the leaves sencha. Theanine is quite different from the polyphenol and catechin antioxidants for which green tea is typically consumed.

I can personally attest to the good feelings you get after a couple cups of green tea. It leaves you with a peaceful feeling without compromising motivation and mental activity.

Bodybuilding and fitness uses

Pre-workout - Green tea is a great alternative to the ECA stack. Yeah I know nothing on the market beats the ECA stack but hear me out. A number of people, including myself do not like how the ECA stack makes us feel. The green tea is great because it does have some caffeine and the theanine really relaxes you mentally but lets you perform physically.

Cutting - Research suggests that supplementing with green tea can **raise your resting metabolic rate by 3%.** In order to get this benefit you must have about 3 glasses a day. If you have a BMR of 2000 or so that means 60 extra calories a day. Why do you see so few obese Asians? It's not the kung-fu. It's the green tea!

All about other teas

All teas come from the same source. The tea plant is a member of the Camellia family (Camellia sinensis). Black tea, oolong tea, and green tea are all derivatives of this one plant.

It is the way the tea is prepared that determines its color. After the tea plant is picked, it is fermented, and then heated to stop the fermentation process. This fermentation process is responsible for the caffeine content of the tea. The longer it is fermented the more caffeine the tea will have. Green tea has the least amount of caffeine of all the teas because it is the least fermented. **The reason why green tea has the most health benefits is because a longer fermentation process destroys many of the beneficial substances in the tea plant.** That is why chugging your Lipton tea is not even remotely comparable to having a cup of green tea. Lipton is made from black tea by the way.

Qualities of tea

There is a huge quality difference in tea. Tea has been compared to wine when it comes to grading. The crap you get when you buy a package of tea at the supermarket and the tea you can get in loose whole leaf form is worlds apart in taste and quality. When selecting tea to be put in bags and sold commercially, manufacturers select the cheapest and lowest quality grade available. The leaves are broken and packed into the small tea bags. Breaking the leaves apart like this degrades the taste and eliminates some of the healthful macronutrients.

The Doctor Says:
Green tea has so many benefits there isn't a good reason for everyone to be drinking it. And its cheap too!

I suggest ordering your tea in whole leaf form. Try to get organically grown green tea in loose-leaf form for maximum benefit. If you do not like the taste of green tea supplementing with green tea extract is always and option.

Green tea summary

Green tea can be a great addition to the fitness enthusiast's arsenal. It is no wonder there is a media blitz telling you green tea is the latest, greatest supplement. But it is no more "the latest supplement" than food is. It's been around for 1000s of years and there are billions of Asians who swear by it.

Ephedrine = a dangerous drug??

If you open a bodybuilding magazine or walk into any given supplement store, you get flooded with the wildest claims about the latest diet supplement pill that will make you lose X amount of pounds a week and turn you into a hulking Greek God in 6 weeks. On the flip side of the coin, we have lawmakers and aggressive media claiming that these are dangerous diet supplement pills. Which are actually just a combination of ephedrine and caffeine and little more in 9 cases out of 10; kill people right and left and should be banned immediately? According to the federal government.

What's up with that? Are they really dangerous, or are they the magic key to ripped abs? The answer is: Yes to both questions - all depending on how you approach the issue. It is true that ephedrine has killed people in extreme cases. It is also true that millions of people use them with little or no side effects.

Ephedrine = death?

As with everything else, too much of anything isn't good for you. Vitamins are great, unless you decide to chug a 100-pill bottle a day. Then you get sick. Not because vitamins are necessarily bad for you, but because you're a moron without common sense who won't read the label.

The same holds true for ephedrine-based diet supplements. It is not for everyone. The labels clearly state that kids, pregnant women, those with high blood pressure, and some other medial conditions should not use them. What is more, the labels usually recommend a low to moderate dosage per day.

Let's ask ourselves: How many of the serious cases used as grounds for banning ephedrine in supplements are caused by:

- Exceeding the recommended dosage.
- Using the product in spite of medical condition.

Unfortunately, I haven't been able to find any statistics for this, but I know that each and every case I've read about was caused by one of the two above.

The Doctor Says:
Ephedrine is a very safe supplement as long as it is used correctly. Overdose on it and it may harm you just like anything taken in excess.

It is my belief that used sensibly we have little to fear from ephedrine. **We must respect the drug for what a powerful substance it is, and always put our health first.** It's like being able to have a beer with your friends once in a while. There's no danger in that as long as you respect alcohol and don't try to drive for a couple of hours afterwards. And recognize the ever-present potential for abuse and alcoholism.

It might sound bizarre to talk about alcohol this way, but it puts a perspective on those who happily swallow ten times the recommended dose of diet pills for weeks on end, and then get surprised when they get sick. In a nutshell: Keep it sane and safe. Then you have little to fear.

Hype and misinformation you need to know about

So let's look at the other side of fence. The supplement manufacturers market their stuff as the greatest thing since sliced bread, trying to put on a facade of scientific mumbo-jumbo. Or using professional bodybuilders in an economic pinch. Or the worst of all, trying to wake your competitive instinct by hinting that you can be the guy kicking sand in the face of the other guys on the beach. Any way you look at it, it's 99% hype and bogus.

The main point is that most of the active ingredients are ephedrine and caffeine, usually with some herb that supposedly imitates the effect of aspirin. **The rest is usually fillers, trying to justify the outrageous claims.** Sure chromium picolinate is good for you, and will help you stay in shape in the long run. It'll work over the next 6-12 months and make you more sensitive to insulin, which translates to less fat storage. Once again, over the long run. It is not some 1-hour magic potion.

The other ingredients are typically herbs and components that created some kind of "revolutionary" study back in the 80s. But later were proven useless for one reason or another. Nonetheless, the manufacturer can claim exceptional potency by quoting that first study filled with crap.

Bottom line: It's almost like buying gas. There's very little difference, if any, between the brands that really counts. What you do want to look out for is con-men who don't deliver the goods. You're paying for high quality, and should expect to receive what's on the label. Be wary of knock-offs that look like a big brand product, but is sold for half the price. Granted, some very well might be legit, but like in the case of creatine: Ask for an independent lab report to verify the claim if you're suspicious.

<u>Vitamins and minerals</u>

The lowdown on antioxidants

As far as muscle growth is concerned, it is important to consider the environment in which we live and the high stress levels that we all face everyday. These two factors lead to an increase in the production of free radicals by the body. The body produces these little troublemakers naturally as we obtain energy from our food in a process called oxidative phosphorylation.

The metabolic process

Essentially, **free radicals destroy tissue in search of electrons; antioxidants sacrifice themselves for body tissue by donating an electron to a free radical.** Therefore, if your body is depleted of antioxidants, then you will have a chaotic event occur inside your body. The production of excess free radicals causes damage to the immune system, the nuclei of cells, blood vessel linkage, and cell membrane stability. This damage from free radicals can be seen as being directly related to the increase in cardiovascular disease, cancer, and autoimmune syndromes.

Vitamin A

Vitamin A is a vitamin that has powerful antioxidant properties. It plays an essential role in the maintenance of the skin and the mucous membranes or internal linings of the body. The maintenance of these two tissues helps to prevent environmental toxins from entering the body. Vitamin A also stimulates the immune system in a number of ways, by producing an anti-tumoral effect, enhancing white blood cell function, and increasing the activity of antibodies.

Beta carotene

Beta Carotene is a pigment that gives carrots, and yellow and red fruits and vegetables their color. The body uses Beta Carotene to make Vitamin A and has been shown to be a very powerful antioxidant. Numerous medical studies have proven its anti-cancer effect in the liver, skin, and lungs. Beta Carotene appears to enhance thymus gland function, which increases interferon production and thus stimulates the immune system. Interferon is a powerful immune stimulator and plays a key role in helping the immune system to fight off viral infections.

Vitamin C

Vitamin C, also known as ascorbic acid, first came to fame by preventing scurvy in the British Navy. Before the discovery of vitamin C, sailors on long voyages were highly susceptible to death due to scurvy because their diets contained less than 60mg of vitamin C per day. The British Navy adopted a ration of lemons and limes for their crews and thus earned the nickname "Limeys." Today, vitamin C is the most popular vitamin supplement in North America because it is a very powerful antioxidant.

Unfortunately, most people only consume the RDA (recommended daily allowance) for vitamin C, which is 60mg; this is only adequate if you want to prevent scurvy. To be used as an antioxidant, high-prolonged doses are required. **As Vitamin C is water-soluble, it does not have a toxic effect.** If you take too much, then the worst thing that can happen is that you may have a mild case of diarrhea. However, drinking sufficient amounts of water will prevent this from happening.

Vitamin C is important because it is used to neutralize free radicals produced by environmental toxins. **Cigarette smokers are well known to be deficient in vitamin C and should be taking 5000mg daily just to neutralize the effect of smoking.** Vitamin C is also an important catalyst for other important physiological reactions that keep the body healthy. A catalyst helps to speed up or helps to produce a physiological reaction. In addition, vitamin C plays a major role in collagen production in connective tissues.

Vitamin E

Vitamin E is known as an anti-aging vitamin and is important in maintaining a healthy reproductive system, increased circulation, and the prevention of heart disease. Vitamin E's role as an antioxidant is to protect cell membranes from damage. As discussed previously, free radicals damage cell membranes that led to premature cell death. Selenium is a trace mineral, which is a primary component of the antioxidant enzyme glutathione peroxidase and works well with vitamin E in preventing cell damage.

ALA

Alpha-Lipoic Acid is used by the body to produce energy in the cell and as an antioxidant. In Germany, Alpha-Lipoic Acid is used as a prescribed drug for the treatment of diabetic neuropathy and AIDS. Diabetes causes changes in the metabolism of the body whereby nerves become damaged, which can lead to blindness, and sensory loss in the extremities. Alpha-Lipoic Acid's antioxidant properties have been researched and shown to protect and heal the nerves from free radical damage.

AIDS research has shown Alpha-Lipoic Acid to help the immune system and to prevent the replication of the AIDS virus. This is accomplished through the antioxidant property of reducing free radical concentrations in the blood.

Pycnogenol and grapeseed extract

Pycnogenol and Grapeseed Extract contain procyanidolic oligomers (PCOs), which come from the flavonoid family of plant extracts. **This family of plants also contains Green Tea, which has been in the news for its anti-carcinogenic properties.** The antioxidant properties of PCOs are their ability to be free radical scavengers. Certain antioxidants work as scavengers to get any free radicals get away from your cells.

You can see that the extra protection we need from free radicals to protect our bodies from various diseases and to prevent muscle breakdown, is readily available in a variety of foods. In addition, I feel that it is certainly warranted to take a potent antioxidant daily in order to reach full health potential and avoid protein breakdown in the body.

Obviously, this is probably way more information than you were looking for. However, I think that it is important to be able to speak intelligently on anything that you are taking as a supplement. You have seen that free radicals are very detrimental to the body. **Through supplementing with antioxidants, you can lower your risk of diseases, disorders, and muscle catabolism.** Remember, through supplementation, it is possible to prevent excessive break down of muscle tissue that is accompanied with a training session and speed up the recovery process too!

A listing of the best ones for you

Vitamin A (carotene) - recommended intake 5000 IU/day

Is used for the formation and maintenance of skin, hair, and mucous membranes. Vitamin A helps with bone and tooth growth. It helps you see in dim light.

Best sources of vitamin A are: yellow and orange fruits and vegetables, green leafy vegetables, fortified oatmeal, liver, and dairy products.

Vitamin B1 (thiamine) - recommended intake 50 mg/day

Helps the body release energy from carbohydrates. Helps with growth and muscle tone.

Best sources of vitamin B1 are: fortified cereals and oatmeal, meats, rice, pasta, whole grains, and liver.

Vitamin B2 (riboflavin) - recommended intake 15 mg/day

Helps the body release energy from protein, fat, and carbohydrates.

Best sources of vitamin B2 are: whole grains, green leafy vegetables, organ meats, milk, and eggs.

Vitamin B3 (niacin) - recommended intake 25 mg/day

Involved in carbohydrate, protein, and fat metabolism

Best sources of vitamin B3 are: meat, poultry, fish, enriched cereals, peanuts, potatoes, dairy products, and eggs.

Vitamin B5 (pantothenic acid) - recommended intake 10 mg/day

Helps in release of energy from fats and carbohydrates.

Best sources of vitamin B5 are: meats, whole grains, legumes, fruits, and vegetables.

Vitamin B6 (pyridoxine) - recommended intake 15 mg/day

Helps build body tissue and aids in metabolism of protein.

Best sources of vitamin B6 are: fish, poultry, lean meats, bananas, prunes, beans, whole grains, and avocados.

Vitamin B12 (cobalamin) - recommended intake 6 mcg/day

Aids cell development, functioning of the nervous system, and the metabolism of protein and fat.

Best sources of vitamin B12 are: meats, dairy products, and seafood.

Biotin - recommended intake 500 mcg/day

Involved in metabolism of protein, fats, and carbohydrates.

Best sources of biotin are: grain products, yeast, legumes, and liver.

Folic acid - recommended intake 1 mg/day

Aids in genetic material development and involved in red blood cell production.

Best sources of folic acid are: green leafy vegetables, organ meats, peas, beans, and lentils.

Vitamin C (ascorbic acid) - recommended intake 3000 mg/day

Essential for structure of bones, cartilage, muscle, and blood vessels. Helps maintain capillaries and gums, aids in the absorption of iron. Helps boost the immune system and is good for reducing muscle soreness after a workout.

Best sources of vitamin C are: citrus fruits, berries, and vegetables

Vitamin D - recommended intake 600 IU/day

Aids in bone and tooth formation, helps maintain heart action and nervous system.

Best sources of vitamin D are: fortified milk, sunlight, fish, eggs, butter, and fortified margarine.

Vitamin E - recommended intake 1200 IU/day

Protects body cells, body tissue, and essential fatty acids from harmful destruction in the body. Helps boost the immune system and is good for reducing preventing some of the side effects from overtraining such as infection and sickness.

Best sources of vitamin E are: multigrain cereals, nuts, wheat germ, vegetable oils, and green leafy vegetables.

Vitamin K - recommended intake 125 mcg/day

Essential for blood clotting functions and helps strengthen bones.

Best sources of vitamin K are: green leafy vegetables, fruit, dairy products, and grain products.

Minerals to maintain in your diet

Calcium - recommended intake 1000 mg/day

Calcium helps strengthen bones, teeth, and muscle tissue. It regulates heartbeat, muscle action, nervous function, and blood clotting.

Best sources of calcium are: dairy products

Chromium - recommended intake 300 mcg/day

Chromium helps with glucose metabolism and it increases the effectiveness of insulin.

Best sources of chromium are: corn oil, clams, whole grains, and brewers yeast.

Copper - recommended intake 3 mg/day

Helps with the formation of red blood cells, bone growth and health. Works with vitamin C to form elasin.

Best sources of copper are: grain products and white potatoes.

Iodine - recommended intake 150 mcg/day

Iodine is a component of hormone thyroxine; it helps in the production of thyroid hormones, which control metabolism.

Best sources of iodine are: seafood and iodized salt.

Iron - recommended intake 30 mg/day

Iron helps with hemoglobin formation. Improves blood quality. Increases resistance to stress and disease.

Best sources of iron are: meats, organ meats, and legumes.

Magnesium - recommended intake 500 mg/day

Helps with acid / alkaline balance. Important in metabolism of carbohydrates and minerals. Can improve strength by increasing protein synthesis.

Best sources of magnesium are: nuts, green vegetables, and whole grains.

Manganese - recommended intake 5 mg/day

Helps with enzyme activation; carbohydrate and fat production; sex hormone production; skeletal development.

Best sources of manganese are: nuts, whole grains, vegetables, and fruits.

Phosphorous - recommended intake 1000 mg/day

Helps with one development and is important in protein, carbohydrate, and fat utilization.

Best sources of phosphorous are: fish, meat, poultry, eggs, and grains.

Potassium - recommended intake 4000 mg/day

Helps with fluid balance. Controls activity of heart muscle, nervous system, and kidneys.

Best sources of potassium are: fruits and vegetables.

Selenium - recommended intake 150 mcg/day

Protects body tissues against oxidative damage from radiation, pollution, and normal metabolic processing.

Best sources of selenium are: seafood, organ meats, meats, and grains.

Sodium - recommended intake 2000 mg/day

Helps regulate fluid balance. Helps regulate acid/base balance in the bloodstream and facilitates active cellular transport across cellular membranes.

Best sources of sodium are: salt.

Zinc - recommended intake 25 mg/day

Involved in digestion and metabolism. Important in the development of the reproductive system. Aids in healing.

Best sources of zinc are: meats, liver, eggs, seafood, and whole grains.

Don't shy away from salt, it can help you

Sodium and its uses are very misunderstood and often-confused health topics. With the media flip-flopping on whether sodium is good or bad for you, it's no wonder why you may be confused.

Sodium will actually help your bodybuilding efforts. Do you want to add mileage to the money you invest in supplements? Simply adding table salt to your daily meals can be extremely helpful in doing so. This "supplement booster" efficiently transports nutrients into your system and, at about $0.50 for a 26-ounce package, is really inexpensive.

Liberally salting your food will help your body transport important bodybuilding nutrients and supplements (like creatine and glutamine) into your muscles more efficiently. No, salting your food won't *cause* high-blood pressure, although excess salt could exasperate high-blood pressure if you already have it.

After getting accustomed to its use, salting your food won't bloat you either. If you drink enough water, your body will routinely flush excess sodium out of your system. If you find yourself looking bloated due to the amount of sodium you are eating, try drinking more water. Keep drinking more water until you find the right amount needed to neutralize or balance out the amount of salt you are eating.

By the way, this strategy is intended for everyone, whether you're a competitive or a non-competitive bodybuilder. Many bodybuilders mistakenly believe they need to carry extra body weight in order to build muscle. It's highly unlikely that an addition of 10 to 30 pounds within a year's period of time would be all quality muscle.

But you say that you are much stronger in the gym with that extra weight? You feel the confidence and certainty the extra body weight gives you improves your training performance and leads to better gains? I agree, but here's a solution, what is more efficient than putting on body fat or adding sodium to your diet?

The Doctor Says:
Depending on how much processed food you eat, you may already have a high amount of salt in your diet. Experiment by adding salt to your food for taste, and then add a little more.

You'll need to experiment with what the right amount is for you, but adding salt to your food, can help you gain an additional 5 to 10 pounds of extra body weight. The extra weight can help you feel stronger, train heavier, prevent injuries, and give you more confidence. **Adding salt to your diet, along with drinking plenty of water, will give you the very same benefits as body fat, but in a much more efficient manner.** Losing the extra water your body carries as a result of adding salt is a process that takes a matter of days. Losing extra body fat is a process that can take months!

Eating a well balanced diet that includes lean meats, poultry, fish, fruits, vegetables, dairy products, and grain products will cover most of your vitamin and mineral needs. You should also take a multivitamin and mineral supplement capsule in the morning with your breakfast and another one in the evening with your dinner. This will ensure that you are getting ample amounts of vitamins and minerals in your daily diet. If you sweat a lot during the day, like during workouts, you should also use a little table salt on your food to help replace lost sodium and prevent muscle cramps.

The dangers of excess body fat

Most people's primary motivation for weight management is to improve their appearance. Equally important, however, are the many other benefits of proper nutrition and regular exercise.

Weight management through reduction of excess body fat plays a vital role in maintaining good health and fighting disease. In fact, medical evidence shows that obesity poses a major threat to health and longevity. The most common definition of obesity is more than 25 percent body fat for men and more than 32 percent for women. **An estimated one in three Americans has some excess body fat; an estimated 20 percent are obese.** Excess body fat is linked to major physical threats like heart disease, cancer, and diabetes.

For example, if you're obese, it takes more energy for you to breathe because your heart has to work harder to pump blood to the lungs and to the excess fat throughout the body. This increased workload can cause your heart to become enlarged and can result in high blood pressure and life-threatening erratic heartbeats.

Obese people also tend to have high cholesterol levels, making them more prone to arteriosclerosis, a narrowing of the arteries by deposits of plaque. This becomes life threatening when blood vessels become so narrow or blocked that vital organs like the brain, heart or kidneys are deprived of blood. Additionally, the narrowing of the blood vessels forces the heart to pump harder, and blood pressure rises. High blood pressure itself poses several health risks, including heart attack, kidney failure, and stroke. About 25 percent of all heart and blood vessel problems are associated with obesity.

The Doctor Says:
The bottom line is: Some fat is healthy and benefits you; excess body fat causes serious health risks, especially in the long term.

Clinical studies have found a relationship between excess body fat and the incidence of cancer. By itself, body fat is thought to be a storage place for carcinogens (cancer-causing chemicals) in both men and women. In women, excess body fat has been linked to a higher rate of breast and uterine cancer; in men, the threat comes from colon and prostate cancer.

There is also a delicate balance between blood sugar, body fat, and the hormone insulin. Excess blood sugar is stored in the liver and other vital organs; when the organs are "full," the excess blood sugar is converted to fat. As fat cells themselves become full, they tend to take in less blood sugar. In some obese people, the pancreas produces more and more insulin, which the body can't use, to regulate blood sugar levels, and the whole system becomes overwhelmed. This poor regulation of blood sugar and insulin results in diabetes, a disease with long-term consequences, including heart disease, kidney failure, blindness, amputation, and death. Excess body fat is also linked to gall bladder disease, gastro-intestinal disease, sexual dysfunction, osteoarthritis, and stroke.

Reducing body fat reduces disease risk

The good news is that reducing body fat reduces the risk of disease. At the University of Pittsburgh, researchers studied 159 people as they followed a weight management program. The subjects were under age 45 and 30-70 pounds overweight. Those subjects who were able to shed just 10-15 percent of their weight and keep it off during the 18-month study showed significant improvement in HDL cholesterol and triglyceride levels, waist-to-hip ratio, and blood pressure. In fact, according to the New England Journal of Medicine, body fat reduction is a more powerful modulator of cardiac structure than drug therapy.

For people with a family history of heart disease, an active lifestyle can slow or stop the process for all but those with serious genetic disorders. Studies by Dr. Dean Ornish, have shown that a comprehensive intervention program that includes regular physical activity, a low-fat diet and a stress reduction program can even reverse the heart disease process.

Evidence also shows that an active lifestyle and its help in reducing body fat is associated with a reduced risk for some types of cancers: prostate for men, breast and uterine cancers for women. Just a few more reasons to get into weightlifting!

In addition, regular physical activity and a low-fat diet are successful in treating non-insulin dependent diabetes (NIDDM); for some patients, it has reduced or eliminated the need for insulin substitutes. In general, regularly active adults have 42 percent lower risk of developing NIDDM.

Gaining fat happens to us naturally

The average American gains at least one pound a year after age 25. Think about it. If you're like most Americans, by the time you're 50, you're likely to gain 25 pounds of fat, or more. In addition, your metabolism is also slowing down, causing your body to work less efficiently at burning the fat it has. At the same time, if you don't exercise regularly, you lose a pound of muscle each year. Consequently, people are not only increasing their body fat stores, increasing their risk of disease, but they're also losing muscle, increasing the risk of injury, decreasing activity performance, and further slowing down metabolism.

Very few Americans exercise in any significant way. The President's Council on Physical Fitness and Sports estimates that only one in five Americans exercises for the healthy minimum of 20 minutes, three or more days a week. In fact, the average American gets less than 50 minutes of exercise per week. Even worse, two out of five Americans are completely sedentary.

Healthy eating and fitness are the best

defenses against being fat

But there is hope. Moderate weight loss, of fat, not muscle, and a healthy and active lifestyle, not dieting; have been found to lower health risks and medical problems in 90 percent of overweight patients. Improving their heart function, blood pressure, glucose tolerance, sleep disorders, and cholesterol levels, as well as lowering their requirements for medication, lowering the incidence and duration of hospitalization, and reducing post-operative complications. **Fit people are also eight times less likely to die from heart disease.**

So, are you willing to be patient and make the changes in your life that will lead to a healthier, happier you? Once you have made the decision to go forward and accept change, the hard part is over. Sure, there is plenty of work to be done, but it really doesn't matter how long this new process takes. If you allow changes to take place over the course of a year, your body will adjust comfortably, and you will be more likely to maintain the healthy lifestyle permanently.

When you begin achieving improvements in energy and physical and psychological performance, the fun and excitement you experience will make the change well worth the effort. Action creates motivation! Good luck: I hope you enjoy all the wonderful benefits of a safe and effective weight management program.

Turning fat into muscle myth

Many health and fitness magazines alike splash the wonderful promise of turning fat into muscle on their covers once in a while. **You simply cannot transform fat tissue into muscle. Muscles mass and fat are two different animals:** Muscle is active tissue that burns calories around the clock even as you sleep, kind of like an engine running in neutral. When you move around, you burn more calories, just like a car will consume more gas the faster you go.

Fat, on the other hand, is just storage of excess energy. It does nothing but sit there with its sole goal in life to be a spare tire around your waist until you put in the effort to burn it off. Bodyfat is not particularly useful except as padding against bumps, as insulation to preserve warmth, and as a convenient surface where you can balance a can of beer while watching the game, as frequently demonstrated by my potbellied neighbor. You need some bodyfat to stay healthy of course, but unless you're walking around with razor-sharp abs and sunken-in, fat-depleted cheeks year-round, you probably have nothing to fear.

Having recognized the difference between the two, let's get down to business: Getting rid of the fat and grow the muscles. It can be difficult to achieve both goals at the same time. The reason for this is that in order to maintain an environment in your body that facilitates fat burn, you must deplete yourself of calories. Growth requires extra calories, much like you'd need extra building material to add a room to your house. In addition, **insulin, which is a key component of growing muscle, is the anti-Christ of fat burn and is released whenever you eat carbohydrates.** How much and how fast depends entirely on the type of carbs, however.

I recommend beginning by trying to pack on the muscle. That means you'll have to eat extra calories, including the extra carbs, and live with the fact that you'll probably gain a few pounds of lard in the process. There's no need to worry about this as long as you keep the increase in bodyfat under control and avoid ballooning like the Pillsbury Doughboy. **Train heavy; eat lots of healthy bodybuilding food (pasta, rice, chicken, lean beef, tuna, oatmeal etc.) but no junk food, candy or alcohol.**

When you've packed on perhaps 5 or 10 pounds of muscle (or whatever your goal was,) switch gears and start the diet. As always, you'll have to keep a daily log of what you eat and carefully adjust your eating patterns so that you eat an average of 500 calories less than you burn each day. Here's where you reap the benefit of having gained the muscle beforehand: Remember the analogy of your muscles being like an engine running in neutral? Muscle burn calories 24/7, and the more mass you have, the more calories are burned without you even having to lift a finger. This in turn translates to a more lenient diet. In other words, if your added muscle mass boosts your natural metabolism by, say 200 calories per day, **that's 200 calories more you can eat and STILL lose bodyfat!** In other words, you'll look better, get to eat more, and will still lose fat at the same rate.

As you diet, you want to keep the protein intake up. Also make sure to keep hitting the weights as you did before; it's your best insurance policy against losing your hard earned muscle mass. The goal at this point is to slowly but surely shave off the fat without sacrificing mass, so take it easy. No sudden changes in eating habits will improve your situation; only worsen it. After a few months you should have lost at least 10-15 lbs of fat, and if you played your cards right, you should have kept most of the gains you made prior to the diet. By taking a little more time and splitting up your two goals, you achieved what you wanted.

The Doctor Says:
During your fat loss training / diet regimen you need to keep up your protein intake. This will help spare the amino acids in your muscles from being consumed and protein foods make you feel fuller so you can keep your total calories low.

<u>**Look for motivation and inspiration**</u>

After the initial novelty of starting a workout program wears off, one problem nearly everyone runs into is lack of motivation. I can personally confirm this just by the membership attrition (drop out) statistics in my health club. 50% of all people who join a health club quit in the first three months. Here's how you can prevent becoming a statistic.

Always be on the lookout for something to motivate and inspire you, anything! Go see a movie, watch a video, read a book or article. Hire a coach or personal trainer. Get a training partner. Think about your goals and write them out repeatedly. Pick a role model of someone you want to look like. Attend a competition. Enter a competition. Hang out with people who motivate you. Ditch the people who don't support you. The list of motivational methods is endless.

Some people ask me, "why bother" with all that positive thinking, goal setting and motivational stuff? They insist that "motivation" doesn't last. I always tell them they're right! Motivation doesn't last, but neither does bathing and you do that every day, don't you? Every day you must ask yourself, "What can I do, find, listen to or watch to get inspired today?" Then follow through. I recently watched a movie called Without Limits, which is the story of Steven Prefontaine, the runner. Even though I'm a bodybuilder and not a runner, that movie got me so motivated I ran to the gym and blasted out a leg workout like never before, smashing through several personal records. I also have the videos of the 1996 Atlanta Olympics narrated by Bud Greenspan. If watching Michael Johnson win his races and accept his gold medals doesn't motivate you, then nothing will.

For the bodybuilders, here's an old motivational stand-by. Watch or re-watch Pumping Iron. For even more inspiration, watch one of Ronnie Coleman's two training videos. That man is a freak! One of the absolute best ways to get motivated is to spend time in serious thought about what you want to accomplish and then write it down.

Set new and bigger goals

If you ever feel unmotivated and you want to get over it, just take a look at your goal list. What? You don't carry a frequently updated, written goal list around with you? Well, I guess we know why you're not motivated don't we?

Goal setting is not an event; it is an ongoing process. When you move up the ladder to intermediate status, the modest goals of a beginner are a thing of the past. "I am walking for 30 minutes three days every week" is a great beginning, but now it's time to move out of the minor leagues.

Goals are the fuel in the fire of motivation. Goals get you out of bed early and into the gym in the morning. Goals keep you on the treadmill for forty-five minutes when you feel like stopping at thirty. In a set of ten reps, goals are what make you push for that eleventh and twelfth rep.

Goals are so much more powerful than you can imagine. Read any book on the subconscious mind, such as "The Power of Your Subconscious Mind" by Dr. Joseph Murphy and you'll begin to understand why goals are so important. If you don't have goals and if you don't have a new set of them every few months, then you're not ready to move up to the next level. **And one last thing, a goal is not a goal if it's not in writing; it's only a wish.**

Read, study and learn

Read one hour a day, five days a week, about training, nutrition, and personal achievement. In three years you will be an expert.

Suppose you only read 30 minutes a day, but you do it every day as a discipline. That's one book every 3 weeks, 18 books per year, and 180 books in ten years. Think about the level of knowledge you'll achieve. I personally read two or three hours a day, I have 700 books in my library and several hundred audio and video programs. I'll miss an hour of sleep before I'll miss an hour of reading. People always ask me how I learned so much about bodybuilding and nutrition. Now you know.

Do you have the power to change?

Do you truly believe that you have the power to change? Doubt can do many things. I had doubt. I told myself I wanted to become lean. Here, "want" was not powerful enough. Why? I did not think that I should become lean, I just wanted to. But I was only hoping and grasping - a part of me did not think it was truly possible. This creates a negative feedback loop. When you only want to succeed, then subtle decisions affect the outcome.

For example, if you are underneath several pounds of iron in the gym and getting ready to push out another rep, but your arms ache so bad you can barely grip the weight, what are you going to do? If you only want to succeed, but don't truly believe that you can, you might decide that the pain is not worth it. So instead of pushing that last rep, you decide to terminate the set and rack the weights. It's okay, it was just one rep, and it wouldn't have been worth it anyway, right?

What am I asking for? I just mentioned moving from "should" to "want" and now I have an issue with "want"! That's right. For certain decisions in your life, it's not enough to want them. You must make them happen. Yes! It's not a possibility, but a certainty. Instead of wanting to obtain your peak physique, understand that you will. When you have made the decision to stop wanting and start creating, then you will cross yet another barrier. When you are underneath that same set of weights, you'll realize that racking them is not an option. Why? Because you will earn your peak physique, so you must get that last rep in. It IS worth it, because **by pushing 110% each and every time, you will reach your goal.**

19 get moving motivators

Studies have shown that carrying groceries, doing yard work, and cleaning your house counts as physical activity. So, while you're not exercising per se, you're at least giving your body some physical benefits. But still you know that this kind of activity isn't going to guarantee a flatter stomach, greater strength, and a longevity boost. So how do find time and energy reach your fitness goals? Here are every-day tips for your inspiration....

1. Take a picture of yourself and have it "morphed" at a photo shop. Want to see how you look 10, 20, 30 pounds heavier? Have the picture people edit the picture in the image you like, then take home copies of it and hang them everywhere you can see it. Harness the power of visualization.

2. Keep a stack of your favorite magazines that you promise yourself you can read only at the gym. If the issues start piling up, you know it's time to schedule a workout.

3. Did you know that not exercising at all is equivalent to smoking a pack of cigarettes every 4 days? (Fear is a good motivator for some.)

4. Your dog. If you want your pooch to enjoy a longer, healthier life, s/he needs to get moving, too. You'll find as both of you get fit, s/he is more enthusiastic, and will give you a challenging workout. If not, YOU give him/her a challenging workout.

5. Work out with your spouse/partner. Not only does it get both of you healthy and strong, but can also spice up your romantic life.

6. Erase YEARS off your body. Chronologically you may be 30, but with regular, vigorous exercise and healthy nutrition, people are going to do a double-take and think you're in your mid-20's. Imagine how awesome you'll feel, when you not only feel younger, but to other people you look younger. Act younger, too.

7. Begin an accomplishments journal. At the end of each day, write down what you've accomplished that day to move you closer toward your fitness and/or life goals. **DO NOT WRITE DOWN WHAT YOU HAVEN'T ACCOMPLISHED.** That doesn't matter. What matters is what you ARE doing; we all need a long-overdue, well-deserved pat on the back on a regular basis.

8. Use the TV. Here's the catch: work out only when your favorite show is on. Or, record your favorite show and work out during that can help time to fly by faster.

9. Hire a personal trainer or coach. If you're having extreme difficulty with motivation, hire a professional to get you to reorganize your life to make taking care of yourself a top priority (which it should be). A good coach or trainer will teach you how to help yourself, without you having to hold someone else's hand, and help you realize that you have the power and ability to do this on your own.

10. Split your workouts. Some recent studies are showing that a split workout can burn more calories than one full workout. So if time's an issue (gee, there's a thought) try getting up 30 minutes earlier in the morning for a short-burst 15 minute workout, then steal another 15-20 minutes at lunch or in the evening.

11. Use your daily planner. You have important commitments scheduled into your planner, right? Volunteer work, doctor appointments, children's activities, etc. Where's EXERCISE?? It's as important a commitment (if not more) than your other activities. Quick tip: mark "EXERCISE" in your planner with a bright colored marker, so it stands out as a reminder to get your butt in gear.

12. **Listen to audio books while you exercise. Self-improvement and motivation books are GREAT here.** You'll feel twice as productive, and highly energized, and the time will fly.

13. Reward yourself. It never ceases to amaze me how hard we are on ourselves when we don't accomplish something, and how hard we are on ourselves when we DO accomplish it.

14. Have kids? Look at their pictures to remind you that you want to be around to share life with them, with plenty of energy. You don't want your 10-year old to be throwing you around the house, do you?

15. Keep a journal of how you feel after exercise. Especially the great workouts. On the days you just don't feel like exercising, look back on the good workout days for some inspiration.

16. See exercise as a stress-releaser. A simple shift in attitude can do wonders for your stress levels. If you've had a long, hard day at work, exercise is something to **look forward to** so you can relieve your stress and revive yourself.

17. Check out the e-mail, chat, or discussion groups on the Internet that deal with fitness, weight loss, diet, exercise, etc.

18. Have young kids? Use the day care at the gym - so there's no excuse about who's going to watch the kids. Or, have a family member(s) or a friend watch them. **So there REALLY is no excuse for not working out.**

19. Look in the mirror. Sometimes that is all you need to trigger you into the lean, fit, and energized mode.

Conclusion

High-intensity for bodybuilding involves the application of maximum effort to build maximum muscle in minimum time. High-intensity training bodybuilders don't waste energy trying out the latest super routines in the muscle magazines. They don't train "instinctively." They generally don't squander training times with pumping exercises. They don't adopt the attitude that performing a few extra sets will make up for earlier sets that were poorly executed.

Instead, successful high-intensity training bodybuilders focus mostly on compound exercises such as the dead lift, squat, bent over row, leg press, and other heavy movements. These bodybuilders endeavor to gradually build their poundages by adding a repetition or so each workout and/or increasing the weight by small increments as often as possible, because they know that **getting stronger on the big movements is the best way to stimulate real gains in size.** They know exactly what exercises and weights they are going to use when they arrive at the gym. They strive to get the most out of every repetition and every set.

High-intensity training bodybuilding comprises the soundest application of the principles of exercise physiology. It's a methodical, disciplined, uncomplicated approach to physique development. If you are a drug-free trainee interested in maximizing your natural bodybuilding potential, **high-intensity training is the fastest route to your destination.**

Keep volume low and intensity high

Some claim that you must do a certain number of sets per body part to induce muscular growth. While it's true that the volume of work performed is a consideration, if volume were the primary stimulus for growth then marathon runners would have massively muscle legs. Instead, a casual observation of distance runners almost always reveals thin legs that appear nearly devoid of appreciable muscle.

Intensity that is, the amount of effort applied to each set, supersedes volume when it comes to producing results. Coupled with the gradual progression in poundage, intensity is the key to growth. In fact, one set performed at 100 percent intensity is far more productive than 10 sets performed at 75 percent intensity.

100 percent intensity means performing a set until you are unable, despite your most aggressive effort, to squeeze out one more repetition with good form. This is also known as training to muscle fatigue or failure. It is simple in concept but difficult in execution. Most trainees who think that they are training to fatigue actually terminate their sets well before reaching true fatigue, particularly when it comes to heavy leg exercises. The mind gives out before the body.

High-intensity training bodybuilding is based upon the notion that muscular growth is the result of the body's effort to protect itself from the stress of training heavy. **The more intense the stress, the greater the body's protective response.** This is why the highest possible intensity, taking each work set to the point of muscular fatigue, is required for the fastest progress.

Pushing each set to muscular failure is the most efficient way to train because it ensures the greatest numbers of muscle fibers are stimulated within the shortest amount of time and with the lowest possible volume of work. The all-or-none principle of muscle fiber recruitment states that a muscle uses only the minimum number of fibers necessary to complete a given task and that those fibers contract with maximal force. As you proceed through a set, the muscle fibers that initially lifted the weight become fatigued, forcing fresh fibers to assist in continuing the set. By the time you reach muscular fatigue, most or all of the target muscle fibers have been exhausted. Training to fatigue also ensures that you use the heaviest possible weight for the given number of repetitions. Both of these scenarios set the stage for the fastest possible growth.

This begs the question: if one set to fatigue is good, aren't two sets better and 10 sets better still? No. Performing an excessive number of sets of the given exercise will not increase intensity, it increases volume. It's essential to understand that the body possesses a limited ability to cope with the demands of any stressor, including exercise. **The right amount of high-intensity training leads to results; too much high-intensity training leads to overtraining.** Needless to say, muscular growth will not occur in an overtrained body.

Train briefly and infrequently

Once you understand that training as hard as possible ensures maximum growth stimulation, the next point to grasp is that training as briefly as possible ensures the body has the resources it needs to provide growth. Bear in mind that the body's first priority after a workout is to recover the energy expended during that workout. Only after the body returns to its pre-workout state will it begin the process of supercompensation or growth. It stands to reason that trainees should **perform the minimum amount of work required to stimulate growth to preserve enough energy to foster the growth process.**

There exists no ideal workout length or set. These parameters vary among trainees, depending upon the individual genetic makeup, training history, and lifestyle. But it's safe to say that if you're training in proper high-intensity training style, one or two sets of any exercise is plenty, with six sets being the maximum one should perform for any single body part. Less is probably better for most people.

In general, two workouts per week or a workout every three to four days is sufficient for most to make progress. This applies to advanced trainees as well as beginners. In fact, advanced trainees may need to workout even less often than beginners because their increased strength and ability to generate more effort places their bodies under greater stress. Whatever frequency you initially choose, you should **add more rest days between your workouts if you find that you're still tired and sore by the time of your next workout** or if you fail to increase poundages/repetitions regularly.

Train for strength

Imagine that you currently bench press a maximum of 250 pounds for eight repetitions. You spend the next 12 months performing continuous tension, muscle confusion, and other alleged muscle building techniques. At the end of the twelve-month period, you can still bench press a maximum of 250 pounds for eight repetitions. How much muscle to think you'll have gained? The answer is none. Yes, none, even after years worth of effort.

That's because a relationship exists between the muscle strength and its size. Sadly, many trainees never comprehend this reality. Instead of making a conscious effort to increase their poundages regularly, they fall into the trap of trying every new technique glorified in the bodybuilding magazines. But because they don't get stronger, they don't get bigger.

Don't be swayed by the throng of so-called bodybuilders who perform set after set of an exercise with the goal of achieving a maximum pump. **A pump has nothing to do with true growth; it is merely a temporary state in which the muscle is engorged with blood.**

If you want to build real, lasting muscle tissue, you must make the muscle stronger. This means training for strength. When you're able to do the target number of repetitions with the given weight, it's time to increase that weight. This increase should be small, about five to ten pounds for leg exercises and 2 1/2 to five pounds on upper body exercises is usually enough.

Most people, when they even bother to increase their weights, make the mistake of increasing them too much. This leads to a rapid deterioration of form. Don't be impatient; overtime, small increases add up to a large increase.

Use an appropriate repetition range

Many authorities believe that hypertrophy can be maximized by repetitions in the range of about 8 to 12. This is a useful principle to follow but, in truth, there can be a significant difference in productive repetition ranges among individuals and among body parts within the same individual.

In general, sets of about five repetitions or less should be avoided by bodybuilders because such low repetitions demonstrate strength rather than build it. In addition, sets of about five repetitions or less at a typical cadence heavily stress the joints and connective tissue without keeping the muscle fibers loaded long enough to provoke growth. Sets of about 15 repetitions or more promote greater metabolic and muscular endurance adaptations rather than strength/growth. **This leaves a usable repetition range for bodybuilding purposes of about 6 to 15.**

A compelling amount of evidence suggests that the lower body responds better than the upper body to higher repetition ranges. As such, it may be best use about 10 to 15 repetitions for lower body work and about 6 to 10 repetitions for upper body work. Experiment with both the upper and lower end of these repetition ranges to discover what works best for you.

Focus on the major muscle groups

If you want to get bigger, you are going to have to pay the price in the form of agonizing effort on exercises that allow you to use relatively heavy weights. The focus should be on compound movements that works several muscle groups at the same time, such as the squat, deadlifts, chin up, bent over row, and bench press. In fact, a very productive routine that stimulates serious growth from head to toe can be built around just these five exercises.

That's not to say that calf raises, arm exercises, and abdominal work should be avoided. They can be part of your program, especially once you're an advanced trainee. Just understand that you'll simulate more biceps growth by doing heavy chin-ups and rows than you will by doing set after set of concentration curls.

The majority of the muscle mass on your body is found in your hips, legs, back, and chest. The only way to gain the pounds of muscular body weight that will accentuate your appearance is by increasing the size of these muscles. **Train the large muscle groups heavy and hard and the smaller groups will gain as well.**

Use proper training style and technique

For best results, it's not enough to lift heavy weights, you must lift them properly. Heaving, thrusting, jerking, and bouncing should be avoided at all costs. As a bodybuilder, your mission in the gym is to exhaust your muscles so that they are forced to rebuild larger and stronger. Weights and machines are the tools you used for that purpose. While you want to lift as much weight as possible for given number of repetitions, you want to do so within the context of proper form.

Jerky and bouncing motions may allow you to lift more weight than you otherwise might be able to handle but such motions minimize the load on the muscles you are trying to work. **Such motions also multiply the stress on your joints and connective tissue, setting you up for injury.**

Some training authorities suggest following a 2 to 4 protocol in which the positive motion takes two seconds in the negative motion takes four seconds. This is fine general advice but what's important to remember is that you want to keep the muscle loaded throughout the entire repetition. Lift the weight with power, precision, and focus; pause for second in the fully contracted position; and lower the weight reasonably slowly while feeling the muscle resist the weight all the way down.

Emphasize recovery more than you think you should

Training provides the stimulus for growth but the growth process does not take place while you train. It takes place later when you rest and especially when you sleep.

Taking an adequate number of days off between workouts is only part of the recovery equation. You must also ensure that your rest days are truly rest days. **If your goal is to add substantial muscle to your frame, minimize your activity level outside the gym.** Playing full-court basketball may be fun but doing so regularly will deplete energy that would otherwise be directed toward recovery and supercompensation. Determine your priorities and act accordingly.

Nor can you afford to frolic until the wee hours of the morning if your dream is to get big. Sleep is critical to the growth process and must not be overlooked. Six hours a night is the bare minimum you should sleep and seven or eight hours is preferable. **Understand that even the most painstakingly devised and religiously followed training program will yield little or no gains if you're sleep deprived.**

Eat well and often

If training serves as the catalyst for growth and sleep provides the opportunity for growth, and food provides the raw materials required for growth.

The ideal eating plan to get big is based around lean protein sources (lean beef, chicken breast, turkey breast, fish, egg whites, and low-fat dairy products), complex carbohydrates (oatmeal, brown rice, yams, and potatoes), fibrous carbohydrates (vegetables and whole fruits), and a small to moderate amount of healthy fats (egg yolks, vegetable oils, nuts, and nut butters). The occasional addition, perhaps a few times weekly, of sweets and fast foods is fine, but keep in mind that a steady intake of sugar and fat laden foods can lead to a rapid accumulation of body fat.

Structure your eating plan to provide five to seven moderate size meals each day. **Smaller, more frequent feedings provide your muscles with a constant supply of the nutrients** they need for growth without promoting excessive fat storage. Such an eating plan will keep your energy level stable and minimize cravings.

Supplements such as protein powers and meal replacements should be viewed as conveniences rather than necessities. Natural food should form the cornerstones of your nutrition program, but when time is short a meal replacement or protein drink is preferable to fast food or no food.

Combine machines and free weights

The arguments in supporting both free weights and machines are loud and long. Free weight supporters claim that the balance required to lift free weights provide a stronger growth stimulus to the muscles and machine lovers point out that machine users can work their muscles harder precisely because they don't have to balance the weight. Free weights are said to be a more natural form of resistance while machines are designed to make up for the inherent shortcomings of barbells and dumbbells.

Each side as valid arguments, so why not get the benefits of both by combining free weights and machines in your program? A very productive routine can be designed around barbells, dumbbells, and whatever machines you have access to.

Keep a daily workout record

Most trainees have no idea where they're going to reach their destination because they don't keep track of where they've been. That is, they don't keep a training diary.

To make the most out of high-intensity bodybuilding, you're going to have to keep records. Don't trust your memory; put your performances on paper. For every work set completed, you should write down the weights used and repetitions obtained. Refer to your training diary during your next training session and try as hard as possible to better your previous performance.

This implies, of course, that the only frequent changes in your routine should be in repetitions and poundages, not exercises. While some variety is reasonable, continually changing exercises doesn't give you the benefit of establishing linear progression from workout to workout, which is the basis for long-term improvement. This does not mean you should use the same exercises for years on end. It only means that you should stick with a given exercise until it ceases to work for you. Leave the so-called instinctive training principle, which states that one should "confuse" the muscles by constantly changing exercises from workout to workout, for those who are more interested in being a Poser than in making progress.

Diet to obtain muscular definition and low bodyfat

While getting bigger is the primary goal of the typical trainee, most serious bodybuilders eventually develop the urge to improve their muscular definition. After all, the source of the unique appearance of bodybuilders, the thing that distinguishes them from just another big person who pumps iron is crisp, sharply delineated musculature.

In truth, training for definition is a fallacy. **Definition is not a quality that can be trained into a muscle; it is nothing more than the absence of fat over a well-developed muscle.** The peaks, valleys, separations, and veins that characterize a detailed physique exist in anyone who has developed a respectable degree of muscle mass. If these muscular details cannot be seen, it's because they are obscured by bodyfat.

The best way to train for definition is to adopt a sensible fat loss plan. Put simply, you'll have to eat less. But you want to eat only a little less, starvation diets burn more muscle than fat. A slight reduction, perhaps 300 to 400 calories daily, should be sufficient to set the fat loss machinery in motion. Aim for a loss of just one pound weekly; more rapid weight loss will quickly eat into your hard earned muscle mass.

The best fat loss diets are based around frequent feedings. Eat five to seven small meals a day consisting of lean protein, a moderate amount of carbohydrates, and a small model fat. While mainstream nutritionists typically promote high carbohydrate eating plans, many competitive bodybuilders find that they get their best fat loss results by consuming a moderate amount of carbohydrates, perhaps 40 percent or less of their calories. These bodybuilders also find a better to taper their carbohydrates as the day goes on by eating starchy carbohydrates for breakfast and lunch and fibrous carbohydrates such as broccoli, a staple source of carbohydrates for bodybuilders, during the late afternoon in the evening.

A moderate amount of cardiovascular activity can assist in fat loss. Whether you choose to run or walk at a fast pace outdoors or indoors on a treadmill, or bike indoors or outdoors, or use one of the numerous cardio machines available at commercial gyms. **Start out by performing the activity two or three times weekly for 20 minutes at a moderate intensity.** Gradually increase the duration and number of cardio sessions. Since excessive cardiovascular work can cut into muscle size, perform the minimum amount of cardio activity required to keep fat loss occurring until you reach her goal. Try not to exceed five 45-minute cardio sessions weekly.

While trying to get lean, your approach to weight training should be the same as when you're striving to add mass: train intensely, briefly, and infrequently. At this point, increasing your volume is an even bigger mistake than it was when you training for size, as a decrease in caloric intake and the inclusion of cardio work makes you more susceptible to overtraining.

What about developing an impressive "six-pack" abdominal region? This again is a matter of eliminating excess body fat through diet and cardio. Performing countless crunches, setups, and leg raises in hopes of bringing out the abs is a waste of time and effort. As your percentage of body fat lowers, your abs will become more prominent. **To display a truly impressive rock hard mid-section, you'll need to lower your percentage of body fat too well under 10 percent**, and undertaking that requires discipline and diligence. **Women would need to drop their percentage of body fat to the low teens.**

Questions and answers

I get bombarded with e-mails from all over the world, from Japan to Argentina, and it's interesting to see how small differences there are, really. Everybody wants to know how to get stronger and more buff. Everybody wants to lose bodyfat. Everybody wants to know if protein drinks really work. The last question is a simple "yes," but the two before that are little bit trickier.

Still, there are some more specific questions that inevitably pop up from time to time. Here are a few of them.

Q: My friend has really peaked biceps while mine are not, while we both curl the same weight. How come? What can I do to increase my peak?

A: Unfortunately, the shape of muscle is largely determined by genetics, so blame mom and dad. However, there are some things you can do. The biceps consists of two separate heads, and by smart training you can develop both to their limit. Don't expect to be able to solely pinpoint one of the two, but you can shift the focus a little. One exercise I have found particularly good for bringing out the peak is bicep curls with a straight barbell, where you hold the bar with a more-than-shoulder-width grip and tuck in your elbows against your sides. Experiment a little to see what works best for you. Start with slightly less weight than usual and do 12-15 reps just to feel where the burn materializes. Then flex your biceps in a classic bicep-pose and use your other hand to squeeze the peak of your biceps. If that's where the lactic acid burn is at, you've found an exercise that will work.

Q: I have a horrible sweet tooth, but I need to get in shape. What can I do to avoid going crazy?

A: Use the window of opportunity immediately after your workouts to have a handful or two of candy. As I've talked about before, that is the one time when you should be eating something sugary to get your body back into an anabolic state again. Make sure to get something sugary though, not fat. Fat has a lot more calories per gram than sugar, and fat will slow down the release of the sugars into your blood stream. Examples of good candy: Jelly beans, sugar babies and reduced fat cookies. Examples of bad candy: Chocolate, candy bars and peanut-butter cups.

Q: You say I should do lat pulldowns to the front rather than behind the neck. Why?

A: To work the lats effectively, you must keep your back slightly arched. By pulling the bar to the front, you're all but guaranteed to keep the arch, while a pull behind the neck lends itself to cheating as you get tired. Thereby you could routinely rob yourself of the benefit from the last few reps of each set without even knowing it. In addition, it's a more natural movement to pull the bar to the front. Your shoulders are at less of a vulnerable angle, and as you get stronger you might avoid cumulative shoulder injuries. This is only true for some people, but the bad news is that you usually don't know if you're one of them until it's too late, so play it safe and assume that you are.

Last but not least, there is an important thing to notice about the lat pulls to the front. You might be tempted to lean back too much when you get tired, thus giving yourself an extra pull. Try to avoid this kind of swaying - sit upright with a lightly arched back, and stay that way throughout the exercise.

Q: What are your thoughts on sports drinks such as Gatorade, Hydra Fuel and such?

A: I don't have any problem with them as long as they're consumed in conjunction with hard and prolonged exercise. Most sports drinks are full of sugar and are formulated to replace lost fluid through sweating, so they're not suitable for drinking with your dinner. In the gym or on a field, they're perfectly fine. Just watch for artificial ingredients. If the drink has a long laundry-list of suspicious-sounding chemicals that you can't even pronounce, pick something else.

Q: My friend is considering buying some steroids, but is concerned about getting ripped off rather than getting the real thing. Is there any web site that can help you identify the legit labels and such?

A: Uh-huh. And I bet your "friend" is about your age and height too, right? Look, here's another reason not to take steroids: It's virtually impossible to know what you're taking. If the crook peddling this dope fills a vial with liquid cleaning agent and slaps a realistic-looking sticker on it, you wouldn't have a clue of what you injected until you woke up in the E.R. If you're lucky, that is. I've seen sites where they promise to show you the telltale signs of counterfeit labels, but guess what? The counterfeiters read the same advice! The bottom line is that all you have to go on is the word of the seller, and, quite frankly, do you think he cares more about your health than his own wallet? Really?

Q: I just can't seem to hit my rear delts properly, and that is getting more and more of a problem as my side and front delts grow. What can I do?

A: Try attaching a handle to the lower pulley on a pulley machine. Then kneel on the floor with your side turned to the pulley. Grab the handle with the hand furthest away from the pulley and lean forward so that you support your upper body with your free hand against the floor. Let the handle pull your other arm so that you feel a good stretch in the rear delt. In other words, if you got your right side facing the pulley, you hold the handle in your left hand while supporting yourself with the right hand on the floor. You should be so far away from the pulley machine that you have resistance even at your most stretched. Then simply pull the handle out to the side as far you can without moving or swaying the rest of your body. The only thing moving should be your shoulder and your arm. This way you can experiment with different angles and slight variations to hit the rear delts 100%.

Q: How important is warm-up, really? I know I'm supposed to do at least 5 minutes on the bike before I hit the weights, but I have very little time...

A: Let me put it this way: If you can "afford" 5 minutes more of watching TV, or 5 minutes of dozing after lunch, or whatever, you'd be better off spending those 5 minutes on a warm-up. Not only do you get your body going so that it utilizes fat for fuel better, it also drastically decreases your risk of injury - especially if you're planning on lifting big.

There's no justification for skipping something that can do so much for your health and safety, unless you're a top-level executive who sleeps 3 hours per night and makes 15-minute appointments to play with your kids on the weekends. If you're a mere mortal like the rest of us, who spends a few hours in front of the tube now and then, you're making an active choice to watch TV instead of looking out for yourself. And by the way, don't you think a single torn muscle, with all the handicaps and rehab it involves, makes up for the time you'd save by skipping the warm-up during your entire life? Play it safe - always warm up.

Q: How come the people in before and after-pictures in the ads always look so much better than I do, no matter how hard I work out, diet, and take the supplements they push?

A: And drinking certain brands of soda doesn't make you an extreme-sporting mega hunk either, even if their ad implies so. Read the fine print. There's always a puny little disclaimer saying something to the effect of: "Mr. Ripped on the picture experienced exceptional results. The typical user may not expect similar results." In plain English, that means they all but admit that while the dude on a picture is a nice fairy tale, the Muscle Fairy will most likely visit not you. The sad truth is that there are no shortcuts. When an ad claims that their product is 3,463% better than the competition, it does not mean you'll gain muscle 3,463% faster. In fact, most scientific claims I've seen are taken out of context. Sure, a certain ingredient in product X may do a lot of good for an 80-year old female diabetic, or help an obese lab rat, but to expect even remotely the same results in a 230 lb, 25-year old male bodybuilder is ridiculous. Yet, they can quote the scientific study and advertise it to create the illusion that the 80-year old woman figures somehow applies to you. It's dirty, but it works. Otherwise they wouldn't keep doing it. Of course, there are honest facts in ads, and there are reputable companies who don't try to scam you with inflated claims, but it's generally easy to spot the difference. Remember: If something sounds too good to be true, it usually is.

Q: I have kind of an embarrassing problem... I don't use steroids, and still I've noticed my pecs are kind of "drooping" when relaxed, making them look like the beginning stages of breasts. I train religiously, I have very little bodyfat, and still I think it keeps getting worse! What's up with this??

A: Don't panic. What you're seeing is probably the effect of too much decline bench pressing. Lately, I've seen a surge the number of people using decline presses, the kind where you lock your legs between two rolls and lay with your head down on a declining bench. This often allows you to use slightly more weight in the bench press, which as we all know is the Holy Grail for 99% of the male gym rats ages 15 to 30. The bad news is; the pectoralis major has a fan-shape, allowing you to train different areas to different degrees. If you do a lot of incline presses, you're weaker compared to the flat press, but you train the upper part of your chest. This gives you a well-balanced, rock-solid look. However, if you train the lower part of your pecs too much, especially if neglecting the upper part, you grow the muscles into looking like a flat-chested dude with beginning bitch tits. Make sense? The muscles will grow according to how you train them, so my advice to you is to stop doing decline presses immediately, and focus on flat and incline presses for a couple of months. When you've balanced out and start feeling comfortable again, you can go back to a normal training routine again - splitting the focus equally between the upper and lower part of the chest.

Q: Why is breakfast so important?

A: When you've been asleep for 8 or so hours, you haven't eaten for at least 8 hours, possibly more like 10 or 11 hours. This means your body is really low on amino acids and carbs, both something you want to have floating around in your body to stay anabolic. The best way to break the starvation of your muscles is to have a hearty breakfast as soon as possible as you wake up. Also, if you work out early in the day, it's extra important to get a lot of carbs with your breakfast, as you'll need it to fuel your workout.

Q: What is the best repetition range for building muscle?

A: At an average repetition cadence (speed), generally 8 -12 reps per set will elicit the greatest gains in lean mass. Sets consisting of less than 6 or 8 reps generally focus on muscle strength, whereas a high number of reps each set targets muscle endurance.

Detailed Answer:

The conventional view that fewer reps in each set equates to more muscle gain is a bit too simplistic. In reality, when one performs sets with very high weight and low reps, the main physiological change is a strengthening of neuromuscular pathways. In other words, high weight/low reps strengthen the brain's ability to activate muscle. However, if we bump up the reps slightly while decreasing the weight as necessary, the muscle tissue will perform more total work, and thus more muscle growth will occur. However, if the reps are increased too high, the main effect will be an increase in muscle endurance.

Through research, it has been determined that the best range for hypertrophy (muscle gain) is roughly between 8-12 reps. As the reps are decreased from this range, the program will elicit greater strength gains will less size. In contrast, more than 12 reps mainly allows for increases in muscular endurance.

Q: Does weight training cause high blood pressure?

A: Natural bodybuilders are among the most fit individuals in athletics. While weight training itself has little effect on cardiovascular health, it does not increase blood pressure in the long term. Although blood pressure does rise during any type of exercise, which is not dangerous for healthy individuals. However, most bodybuilders also engage in cardiovascular exercise, which is well established for decreasing blood pressure.

Also, natural bodybuilders tend to be very lean; not only on the "outside," but also on the "inside," as they tend to have less fatty plaque lining artery walls, and are therefore at a reduced risk for atherosclerosis. Further, the "large heart syndrome" that many purport as a result of weight training has not been proven in research.

Q: Is it possible to gain muscle strength or muscle endurance without gaining muscle size?

A: It is possible to gain strength without increasing muscle size (hypertrophy). Similarly, it is possible to enhance muscle endurance without hypertrophy. However, it may be difficult to train for both goals at the same time.

- Training for muscle endurance is generally achieved through high repetitions and lighter weights.
- To train for strength while minimizing gains in muscle mass, it is advisable to perform low repetitions per set, using explosive movements (short concentric contractions) while lowering the weights under control. Be sure to be adequately warmed up before starting into the working sets.

Detailed Answer:

Training for strength over size is largely attained through manipulating the neuromuscular system (brain-muscle connection); that is, strengthening the nervous system as a muscle "activator". As a protective mechanism for the body, the central nervous system has safeguards in place that shut down muscle activity when the muscle attempts to work at too high an intensity.

Specifically, one of these systems works through an organelle found in tendons of muscle, which shuts down muscle activity when it senses that there is too much strain on a muscle. Also, for the untrained individual (or somebody who rarely lifts very heavy weights), the connection between muscle and brain may be relatively weak. To train the neuromuscular connection, it is advisable to perform low repetitions per set, using explosive movements (short concentric contractions) while lowering the weights under control.

Be sure to be adequately warmed up before starting into the working sets. Although muscle fiber density may increase from this type of training, hypertrophy is minimized since high resistance/low rep training does not elicit changes in extra-fibril structures (blood vessels, organelles like mitochondria). At the same time, strength gains will be evident through neuromuscular manipulation.

Training for muscle endurance is generally achieved through high repetitions and lighter weights. With this type of training, the major change to the muscle is the ability to manage metabolic waste, and fuel utilization. For example, the muscle is better able to utilize lactate as a fuel rather than allow it to minimize muscle performance.

Also, more efficient fuel sources such as fats make up a larger portion of the muscle's fuel. Rather than carbohydrates which tend to promote metabolic waste accumulation. Note, however, that some of these changes include increased capillary (and blood vessel) density and mitochondria, changes that reduce muscle density. Nevertheless, these changes will not cause a significant increase in muscle size.

Since these two goals require quite different methods of training, a good approach may be to periodize your training. That is, train for muscle endurance for 3-4 weeks, and then switch to a training program geared towards building muscle strength.

Q: What is meant by the term Basal Metabolic Rate?

A: Basal Metabolic Rate (BMR) or basal metabolism represents the minimal energy expended to keep a resting, awake body alive. This requires about 60-70% of the total energy use by the body. The processes involved include maintaining a heartbeat, respiration, temperature and other functions. It does not include energy used for physical activity or digesting foods. Basal metabolism accounts for roughly 1 kcalorie/kilogram (2.2 lbs.)/hour. I use the term 'roughly," due to the fact that the amount of energy used for basal metabolism depends primarily upon lean body mass.

Q: What causes delayed onset muscle soreness?

A: The cause for delayed onset muscle soreness (DOMS) has been debated at length by exercise physiologists, and is still not fully understood. Mechanisms for theories proposed in the past have included lactic acid buildup, torn tissue, muscle spasm, and connective tissue damage. Of these, the lactic acid buildup theory, and spasm theory have largely been discounted by exercise physiologists. Currently, the most accepted theory for DOMS seems to be muscle/connective tissue damage due to mechanical forces on the muscle and connective tissue.

Q: I heard that exercising on an empty stomach leads to losses in lean body mass. Should I really be exercising on an empty stomach?

A: There are benefits to working out on an empty stomach, and different benefits when one works out after eating. Ultimately, one should choose the method based on their fitness goals. As a rule of thumb, it may be best to perform workouts on an empty stomach if one's main goal is bodyfat loss. However, if one is only concerned with gaining lean mass, eating 30-60 minutes before a workout may be a good idea.

For people looking to lose bodyfat while increasing muscle mass at the same time, it may be best to take advantage of the key benefits of each method. For example, one could try working out on an empty stomach some days, and eat 30-60 minutes before working out on other days (i.e. eat before resistance exercise sessions; do not eat before cardio). Following is a detailed breakdown of the benefits and drawbacks to each method:

Eating 30-60 minutes before a Workout

Benefits:

- Maximizes liver and muscle glycogen, a fuel stored in muscle that is necessary for intense exercise (assuming that the meal is balanced).
- Prevents the breakdown of muscle tissue (by preventing the secretion of the hormone cortisol).
- Allows for longer duration workouts.
- May increase secretion of growth hormone (particularly with exercise that elicits high lactate production, like intense cardio) therefore greater utilization of fat as fuel, free fatty acid (FFA) release, and protein synthesis.

Drawbacks:

- Suppresses FFA release from fat stores (due to the presence of insulin).

• Excess insulin (which easily occurs through eating too many calories or high glycemic foods) may cause hypoglycemia, leading to depleted muscle glycogen stores therefore exerciser "crashes".

Exercise on Empty Stomach

Benefits:

• Increases FFA availability in blood therefore increases the amount fats burned as energy.

• May increase secretion of growth hormone (particularly with exercise that elicits high lactate production, like intense cardio) therefore greater utilization of fat as fuel, FFA release, and protein synthesis (note that this is an unresolved issue, as it contradicts the bullet above).

Drawbacks:

• Increased production of cortisol therefore leads to the breakdown of muscle tissue.

Q: On certain training days such as when I do back and biceps together, sometimes it is difficult to hold onto the bar because of forearm fatigue. Is there anything I can do to correct this?

A: Forearm strength is often a limiting factor, especially when handling heavy weights vertically such as pull-ups or deadlift. Chalk, sticky pads, or weightlifting straps can help with handling the load when necessary, however, as a rule of thumb, it is best to work through this discomfort since these very activities are some of the best exercises for developing the forearms and building grip strength. On the contrary, straps and chalk should always be used.

When to use straps and chalk:

1. Your ability to hold the weight compromises the safety of the movement, or

2. Lack of grip strength limits your ability to strengthen/develop the target muscle effectively.

Q: I have had a cold the past couple of days and was wondering if it is a good idea to still exercise?

A: You may think it is a good idea not to engage in vigorous exercise when you have the sniffles. However, a new study suggests that if you are well enough to get out of bed, you are probably well enough to get a workout. Researchers at Ball State University in Indiana found that exercising does not delay recovery or worsen symptoms of the common cold.

In the study, 34 moderately fit folks, ages 18-29, were assigned to an exercising group, while 16 additional people of similar age and fitness level were assigned to a non-exercising group. Then both groups were inoculated with a virus to produce upper respiratory illness. The exercising group worked out at 70% of maximum heart rate for 40 minutes per day, every other day.

Researchers collected used facial tissues and administered symptom questionnaires every 12 hours to gauge the progress of the illness and its symptoms. After ten days, analyses of symptoms were similar between the exercising and non-exercising groups. So while you may feel like scaling down your routine if you are feeling under the weather, there seems to be no reason to skip it altogether.

Q: I've heard the terms "concentric and eccentric contractions." What do these mean?

A: A concentric contraction occurs during the lifting phase of an exercise, when the muscle shortens or contracts. For example, when you lift the weight in a bench press, pressing it from your chest to the lock-out position, that is the concentric, or "positive," phase of the exercise. An eccentric contraction occurs during the lowering phase of an exercise, when the muscle lengthens. For example, lowering the weight to your chest during the bench press is the eccentric or "negative," portion of the exercise.

Q: What can I do about 'stretch marks' that appear after I've been weight lifting and gaining size and strength?

A: If you are weight training and gaining some size and muscularity, chances are you will begin to develop stretch marks. This is, to a certain extent, unavoidable. You may minimize their development, however, through the application of a topical antioxidant cream that contains collagen. Regular application of this type of lotion/cream will increase skin elasticity, and thus diminish the formation of stretch marks, but it may not fully prevent their development.

Q: What can I do to prevent muscle cramping?

A: Muscle cramping occurs when a muscle continues to contract, and cannot seem to "let go". The painful sensation one feels is caused by muscle fatigue, and waste products like lactic acid that build up in the muscle. Although the cause of muscle cramps is not entirely understood, a number of factors seem to be involved, including hydration level, electrolyte balance, training history, and chronically tight muscles.

Some factors that may increase muscle cramps:

1. Training history seems to be the most important factor. Exercise beyond an accustomed limit (longer duration, or intensity) will often brings on muscle cramps. However, through regular training, one tends to experience muscle cramps less frequently.

2. Make sure that you are drinking enough water - 10 glasses of water daily (at least 10 oz. each), or if you care to be more precise, 0.6oz/water/lb. of bodyweight. Increase this amount if you consume caffeine. For each cup of coffee, tea, or soda you take in, please be sure to add an additional 10 oz glass of water for each.

3. Through sweating (especially in a hot environment), one tends to lose electrolytes like sodium, potassium, and magnesium. Normally these are replaced in the diet. However, prolonged exercise (longer than 1 hour) in hot environments may create a need for mineral replenishment. Try adding a bit of salt to your foods, and take a multivitamin/mineral supplement and see if this makes a difference.

4. Lastly, tight muscles are best addressed by stretching before and after every workout. Stretching allows more nutrients, blood, etc. into the muscle, and allows you to dispose of waste materials more easily due to increased blood flow.

Q: What is the current theory on using a weight belt? Should I or shouldn't I use one?

A: Weight belts are a handy tool for helping to protect your back on those lifts that may stress it, but that does not mean you should use them on every lift for every rep. When you do an intense exercise that involves the back, such as squats, it would seem logical that you would want that safety precaution in place at all times.

In doing so, however, you may predispose yourself to an injury by taking the muscles that would ordinarily act as natural back supports out of the equation. Essentially, when you are doing a squat, your primary focus in terms of strength is your leg muscles. What most people don't realize is that you are also simultaneously strengthening your back support muscles; abdominals, lower back, obliques, etc.

When you wear a belt, you take those muscles (to a lesser or greater extent depending upon form) out of the chain, and as such they do not get strengthened to the same degree as do your leg muscles. What this may do in the long run is create an imbalance in the body in terms of overall support and equilibrium, which as you continue to grow stronger and use more weight, may increase the risk of injuring yourself in one way or another.

Perhaps the best way of looking at these muscles is to consider them a chain, and as you know, a chain is only as strong as its weakest link. As such, if you're going to strengthen any part of the chain, you better strengthen the whole chain to keep yourself safe and prevent injuries. When would you want to use a belt? Usually, the only time to use a belt is when you are attempting a maximal lift; anywhere from 4 - 6 reps of a challenging weight that involves back support and all-out effort. At all other times, it's a good idea to simply use good form and have a competent spotter on these exercises.

Q: I have been told all of my life that you have to work out at least 30 to 35 minutes in order to begin burning fat. Is there any scientific data you can provide to prove that the 20-minute aerobic solution does in fact burn fat?

A: When trying to lose bodyfat, the duration of the workout is less important than total calorie balance (total calories burned). To lose fat, it is necessary to achieve a calorie deficit. That is, the number of calories you burn must be greater than the number of calories you ingest. Cardiovascular exercise helps you to create this calorie deficit by burning excess calories. Although you can burn calories at any workout intensity, it is most efficient to work at a high-intensity for shorter periods of time compared to long-duration workouts.

For example, working at a high-intensity, one can burn up to 50% more calories in a shorter period of time. More importantly, post workout, you continue to burn calories at an elevated rate up to 142% more than low-intensity aerobics within the first hour following the cardio session. What's more, this elevation in metabolism lasts up to 48 hours post workout, an effect not achieved with low-intensity exercise. The bottom line is that while low-intensity, long-duration exercise is effective for fat loss; typically one sees better results using a high-intensity protocol. Plus, this type of training is more efficient since once spends less time in the gym, but typically experiences better results.

Q: I typically run outdoors, but when it's hot and humid, I head to the treadmill. Does running on the treadmill burn fewer calories?

A: If you're running at speeds under 9 miles an hour (a very fast 6:40-minute-mile pace), treadmill running burns about the same number of calories as running outdoors. But if you run faster than 9 mph, you'll burn fewer calories on the treadmill. The difference can be up to 8 percent because you don't have to overcome wind resistance and because the treadmill belt does propel you along a bit.

Q: A year and a half ago, I started running 5 miles on a treadmill six days a week and lifting weights three times a week. The results have been fabulous; a 74-pound weight loss, a huge drop in blood pressure and an enormous surge in self-esteem. But now my knees ache, especially when I walk downhill. Is this a result of running? What can I do about the pain?

A: Six days a week of high-impact training such as running is very hard on the body, especially the knees. Substituting a low-impact activity such as biking, swimming or the elliptical trainer once or twice a week is much healthier.

Most likely you're experiencing patella-femoral syndrome, also known as pain behind the kneecap. Running, especially on hard surfaces, increases the pressure of the patella (kneecap) on the femur (thighbone) when you bend and straighten your knee.

Q: Is it easier for a man to get six-pack abs than for a woman to?

A: Yes. The appearance of defined, rock-hard ab muscles is possible only if the abs are highly trained and there is very little fat on top of them. On average, women have more total body fat than men, and proportionally they nave more subcutaneous fat. What's more, it's easier for men to lose body fat than it is for women, partly due to hormonal differences. If you put men and women on the same exercise and diet program, men will lose more weight on average. Of course, not every man will lose more fat than every woman will. There are exceptions; some women can achieve a six-pack without tremendous work, and some men have no chance of ever having sleek abs.

The bottom line, don't get frustrated if you can't achieve that six-pack. It may not be a matter of lacking willpower. It could be just a matter of genetic and gender destiny.

Q: I have a friend who does a 5- to 10-minute warm-up on a treadmill, then lifts weights, then does 20 more minutes of cardio. Does her warm-up really count as cardlo? I've heard you need to do 15 consecutive minutes to get benefits.

A: A 5- to 10-minute warm-up certainly would count. Since a warm-up is performed at a low intensity, you won't burn as many calories those first few minutes. But that doesn't mean you're not benefiting. Most people don't need more than two or three minutes to get their heart rate up to the lower end of their target zone. At the lower end of the zone — about 60 percent of your maximum heart rate — your body is working hard enough to achieve health and fitness benefits.

There is no research establishing the minimum number of consecutive minutes necessary to "count," but plenty of research has established the benefits of short cardio bouts.

Of course, if you are training for an endurance event such as a 10k or marathon, 10 minute workouts aren't going to cut it. But for general health and fitness you can break it down, research shows tremendous benefits from performing 15 10-minute exercise bouts per week, including cardio exercise, strength training and stretching.

Q: What happens if I go over my target zone for fat burning?

A: You will burn glycogen (blood glucose), which is fine. The problem, however, is that unless you are a highly trained athlete, you don't have high amounts of glycogen stored in your muscles cells and other storage areas. In this case, cortisol, one of the hormones secreted with exercise begins to break down muscle tissue to transform it into glucose so you can continue to exercise/survive. This process is commonly known as "gluconeogenisis," or the new formation of glucose by breaking down muscle.

Q: Why are strong abdominal muscles so important?

A: A strong mid-section will help support the lower back (lumbar spine). It also helps transfer strength and power from the upper body to the lower. In general, the abdominal muscles, lower back, and pelvic region is called the "core." What you need to strive for is "core stability." When the hip flexor muscles are too tight, it causes inflexibility and forward pelvic tilt. Weak abdominals and a tight lower back will create an excessive arch in the lower back known as "sway back." When an imbalance is present in this area, the result can be pain, poor energy transfer in sports, and general body discomfort. Over time, the result can be spinal segments that lip, spur, and even fuse.

Q: How important is massage therapy to an athlete?

A: In one word "VITAL". Massage does the following: reduces stress, decreases recovery time, promotes healing, increases performance, increases speed, releases toxins and it feels oh, so good! Make sure your massage therapist known your tolerance for pain, what type of massage you've experienced, and your intended benefit from the massage.

Q: Should I stretch before or after I workout with weights?

A: Both. Prior to any stretching, a general warm-up should take place. A bike, rower, treadmill or stepper is fine. This is to heat the body's core temperature. Once the core is warm, perform some moderate intensity stretches. Make certain the entire body is stretched, however spend a little extra time on the specific area you intend on training first. After you finish your lifting routine, you body will be very warm and better able to stretch more deeply. This is the time to gently increase the intensity of your stretching.

Q: If I'm very over weight, should I still lift weights? I don't want to bulk up any more.

A: You absolutely should lift weights. It doesn't need to be your focus, but it needs to be included in your complete program. In most cases, weight training is not cardiovascular in nature. This means your body will not use fat as a primary source of energy while lifting weights. However, weight training does make your body better at consuming calories throughout the day. Because a muscle requires more energy to maintain its structure as compared to fat, your body must use (burn) more calories to maintain that muscles integrity. Aside from all this, if you don't maintain or build muscle as you lose weight, you will become what is known as a "thin, fat person." This is a slightly built person who has no muscle mass.

Q: Is there a difference between types of creatines that are currently available?

A: As some people are aware, you can now find creatine on the market in three forms: phosphate, citrate, and monohydrate. My feeling is that the phosphate variety is not easily absorbed by the body and for this reason will not yield effective and substantial results. The citrate variety seemed to be catching on for a time, but again the research is sketchy here. In fact, nearly all the positive clinical studies that have been done on creatine have utilized the monohydrate form, and this is the only form that I currently recommend.

Q: My doctor told me I am allergic to wheat and dairy products. How could this be? Is there a test or a way to really find out if I am allergic?

A: I think the only way you can find this out is by omitting all forms of those foods from your diet for at least a week, then adding the food back and seeing if your symptoms return. Also, since both wheat and dairy products are found in so many foods, you'll have to read the labels of processed foods especially carefully.

Q: I love chocolate. Is it really bad for you? How much can I eat without sabotaging my healthy eating plan?

A: Chocolate isn't all bad. In fact, chocolate is rich in antioxidants called phenolics, the same compounds in red wine that seem to offer protection against heart disease. And cocoa butter, the fat in chocolate, does not appear to be so bad for your heart and arteries. Its principal saturated fat, stearic acid is converted by the body into oleic acid, a heart-healthy monounsaturated fat also found in olive oil. Pick chocolate made with cocoa butter rather than unhealthy fats such as palm and coconut oils. This means look for cocoa to appear in the ingredients before sugar.

Q: I seem to be addicted to sweets. How do you suggest I stop eating foods high in sugar?

A: Taming your sugar cravings could be a matter of slowly reeducating your tastebuds or learning to feel satisfied with less. If you slowly cut back on sweets, you will find that healthy sweet foods taste exceptionally sweet - fresh strawberries, frozen grapes, mangoes, dried unsweetened cherries. Treats like these will satisfy your sweet tooth if you take the time to eat them with full attention to taste, aroma, and presentation.

Q: What are the pros and cons of eating farm-raised salmon instead of salmon from the wild? I've heard farmed salmon is not a good source of omega-3 fatty acids because of what the fish are fed.

A: I always choose wild salmon over farmed salmon. Flesh from most pen-raised salmon may be lower in beneficial omega-3 fatty acids and higher in harmful saturated fats than that from their wild cousins - a consequence of what they are fed. And worst of all, is that the under exercised muscles of salmon reared in cages produce a soft, bland-tasting fish that just doesn't stand up to the wild version. The product label will tell you whether or not the fish was farmed.

Q: What is your take on alpha-lipoic acid?

A: Alpha-lipoic acid (ALA) has a number of admirable qualities including the unique ability to work nearly anywhere in the body. It also appears to be safe, readily converts into a useable form, and neutralizes many different kinds of free radicals. This tiny molecule recycles antioxidants such as vitamin C and E, prolonging their effectiveness.

Terms and definitions

AEROBIC EXERCISE

Prolonged, moderate-intensity work that uses up oxygen at or below the level at which your cardiorespiratory (heart-lung) system can replenish oxygen in the working muscles. Aerobic literally means with oxygen, and it is the only type of exercise, which burns body fat to meet its energy needs. Bodybuilders engage in aerobic workouts to develop additional cardiorespiratory fitness, as well as to burn off excess body fat to achieve peak contest muscularity. Common aerobic activities include running, cycling, swimming, dancing, and walking. Depending on how vigorously you play them, most racquet sports can also be aerobic exercise.

ANABOLIC DRUGS

Also called anabolic steroids, these are artificial male hormones that aid in nitrogen retention and thereby add to a male bodybuilder's muscle mass and strength. These drugs are not without hazardous side effects, however, and they are legally available only through a physician's prescription. Steroids are available in most gyms via the black market, but it is very dangerous to use such unknown substances to increase muscle mass.

ANAEROBIC EXERCISE

Exercise of much higher intensity than aerobic work, which uses up oxygen more quickly than the body, can replenish it in the working muscles. Anaerobic exercise eventually builds up a significant oxygen debt that forces an athlete to terminate the exercise session rather quickly. Anaerobic exercise, the kind of exercise to which bodybuilding training belongs, burns up glycogen (muscle sugar) to supply its energy needs. Fast sprinting is a typical anaerobic form of exercise.

ANDROGENIC DRUGS

Androgenics are drugs that simulate the effects of the male hormone testosterone in the human body. Androgens do build a degree of strength and muscle mass, but they also stimulate secondary sex characteristics such as increased body hair, a deepened voice, and high levels of aggression. Indeed, many bodybuilders and power lifters take androgen to stimulate aggressiveness in the by resulting in more productive workouts.

BALANCE

A term referring to an even relationship of body proportions in a man's physique. Perfectly balanced physical proportions are in a much-sought-after trait among competitive bodybuilders.

BAR

This is the steel shaft that forms the basic part of barbell or dumbbell. These bars are normally about one inch thick, and they are often encased in a revolving metal sleeve.

BARBELL

Normally measuring between four and seven feet in length, a barbell is the most basic piece of weight-training and bodybuilding equipment. Indeed, you can train every major skeletal muscle group in your body using on a barbell. There are two major and types of barbells used for exercise in common use, adjustable sets; in which you can easily add or subtract plates by removing a detachable outside collar held in place on each side by a set screw. And fixed barbells; in which the plates are either welded or bolted permanently in place. Fixed weights are arranged in variety poundages on long racks in commercial bodybuilding gyms, the approximate poundage for each one painted or etched on the bar. Fixed weights relieve you of the problem of changing plates on your barbell for each new exercise. While fixed barbells and dumbbells are normally found in large commercial gyms, adjustable barbell and dumbbell sets are more frequently used at home.

BASIC EXERCISE

This is a bodybuilding exercise, which stresses the largest muscle groups of your body (e.g., the thighs, back, and/or chest), often in combination with smaller muscles. You will be able to use very heavy weights in basic exercises in order to build great muscle mass and physical power. Typical basic movements include squats, bench presses, and deadlifts.

BENCHES

A wide variety of exercise benches is available for use in doing barbell and dumbbell exercises either lying or seated on a bench. The most common type of bench, a flat exercise bench, can be used for chest, shoulder, and arm movements. Incline and decline benches (which are angled at about 30-45 degrees) allow movements for the chest, shoulder, and arms.

BIOMECHANICS

The scientific study of body positions, or form, in sport. In bodybuilding, biomechanics studies body form when exercising with weights. When you have good biomechanics in a bodybuilding exercise, you will be safely placing maximum beneficial stress on your working muscles.

BMR

The basal metabolic rate is the speed at which your resting body burns calories to provide for its basic survival needs. You can elevate your BMR and more easily achieve lean body mass through consistent exercise, and particularly through aerobic workouts.

BODYBUILDING

A type of weight training applied in conjunction with sound nutritional practices to alter the shape of one's body. In the context of this book, bodybuilding is a competitive sport nationally and internationally in both amateur and professional categories for men, women, and mixed pairs. However, a majority of individuals uses bodybuilding methods merely to lose excess body fat or build up a too thin part of the body.

BURN

This is a burning sensation that you feel in the muscle that you are training. This burn is caused by a rapid buildup of fatigue toxins in the muscle and is a good indication that you are optimally working a muscle group. The best bodybuilders consistently forge past the pain barrier erected by muscle burn and consequently build very massive, highly defined muscle.

BURNS

A training technique used to push a set past the normal failure point, and thereby to stimulate it to greater hypertrophy. Burns consist of short, quick, bouncy reps 2-4 inches in range of motion. Most bodybuilders do 8-12 burns at the end of a set that has already been taken to failure. They generate terrific burn in the muscles, hence the name of this technique.

CARDIORESPIRATORY FITNESS

This is the physical fitness condition of the heart, circulatory system and lungs that is indicative of good aerobic fitness.

CHEATING

A method of pushing a muscle to keep working far past the point at which it would normally fail to continue contracting due to excessive fatigue buildup. In cheating you will use a self-administered body swing, jerk, or otherwise poor exercise form once you have reached the failure point to take some of the pressure off the muscles and allow them to continue a set for two or three repetitions past failure.

CHINNING BAR

A bar attached high on the wall or gym ceiling, on which you can do chins, hanging leg raises, and other movements for your upper body. A chinning bar is analogous to the high bar male gymnasts use in national and international competitions.

CIRCUIT TRAINING

A special form of bodybuilding through which you can simultaneously increase aerobic conditioning, muscle mass, and strength. In circuit training, you will plan a series of 10-20 exercises in a circuit around the gym. The exercises chosen should stress all parts of the body. These movements are performed with an absolute minimum of rest between exercises. Then at the end of a circuit, a rest interval of 2-5 minutes is taken before going through the circuit again. Three-five circuits would constitute a circuit-training program.

CLEAN

This movement consists of raising a barbell or two dumbbells from the floor to your shoulders in one smooth motion to prepare for an overhead lift. To properly execute a clean movement, you must use the coordinated strength of your legs, back, shoulders, and arms.

COLLAR

A clamp is used to hold plates securely in place on a barbell or dumbbell bar. The cylindrical metal clamps are held in place on the bar by means of a setscrew threaded through the collar and tightened securely against the bar. Inside collars keep plates from sliding inward and injuring your hands, while outside collars keep plates from sliding off the barbell in the middle of an exercise.

CUT UP (OR CUT)

A term used to denote a bodybuilder who has an extremely high degree of muscular definition due to a low degree of body fat.

DEFINITION

The absence of fat over clearly delineated muscular movement. Definition is often referred to as "muscularity," and a highly defined bodybuilder has so little body fat that very fine grooves of muscularity called "striations" will be clearly visible over each major muscle group.

DENSITY

This is the hardness of the muscle, which is also related to muscular definition. A bodybuilder can be well defined and still have excess fat within each major muscle complex. However, when he has muscle density, even this intramuscular fat has been eliminated. A combination of muscle mass and muscle density is highly prized among all competitive bodybuilders.

DIPPING BAR

Parallel bars set high enough above the floor to allow you to do dips between them, leg raises for your abdominal, and a variety of other exercises. Some gyms have dipping bars, which are angled inward at one end; these can be used when changing your grip width on dips.

DIURETICS

Sometimes called "water pills," these drugs and herbal preparations remove excess water from bodybuilder's system just prior to a show. This reveals greater muscular detail. Harsh chemical diuretics can be quite harmful to your health, particularly if they are used on a chronic basis. Two of the side effects of excessive chemical diuretic use are muscle cramps and heart arrhythmias (irregular heart beats).

DUMBBELL

Essentially, a dumbbell is a short-handled barbell (usually 10-16 inches in length) intended primarily for use with one in each hand. Dumbbells are especially valuable when training the arms and shoulders, but can be used to build up almost any muscles.

EXERCISE

Movements such as a seated pulley row, barbell curl, bench press, or seated calf raise, etc that you perform in your workouts.

EZ-CURL BAR

A special type of barbell used in many arm exercises, but particularly for standing EZ-bar curls wherein it removes strain from your wrists. An EX-curl bar is also occasionally called a "cambered bar." Albert Beckles, one of the sport's most successful professionals from the 1980's, whimsically calls this piece of equipment a "wiggly bar" because of its shape.

FAILURE

That point in an exercise, which you have fully fatigued your working muscles. They can no longer complete an additional repetition of a movement with strict biomechanics. You should always take your post-warm-up sets at least to the point of momentary muscular failure, and frequently past that point.

FLEXIBILITY

A suppleness of joints, muscle masses, and connective tissues, which lets you, move your limbs over an exaggerated range of motion, a valuable quality in bodybuilding training, since it promotes optimum physical development. Flexibility can only be attained through systematic stretching training, which should form a cornerstone of your overall bodybuilding philosophy.

FORCED REPS

Forced reps are a frequently used method of extending a set past the point of failure to induce greater gains in muscle mass and quality. With forced reps, a training partner pulls upward on the bar just enough for you to grind out two or three reps past the failure threshold.

FORM

This is simply another word to indicate the biomechanics used during the performance of any bodybuilding or weight-training movement. Perfect form involves moving only the muscles specified in an exercise description, while moving the weight over the fullest possible range of motion.

FREE WEIGHTS

Equipment such as: Barbells, dumbbells, and related equipment. Serious bodybuilders use a combination of free weights and such exercise machines as those manufactured by Nautilus and Universal Gyms, but they primarily use free weights in their workouts.

GIANT SETS

Performing a series of 3-5 exercises, done with little or no rest between each movements, and a rest interval of 3-4 minutes between each giant sets. You can perform giant sets for either two antagonistic muscle groups or a single body part.

HYPERTROPHY

This means increase in muscle mass and an improvement in relative muscular strength. Placing an "over-load" on the working muscles with various training techniques during a bodybuilding workout induces hypertrophy.

IFBB

The International Federation of Bodybuilders, the gigantic sports federation founded in1946 by Joe and Ben Weider. With more than 120 member nations, the IFBB proves that bodybuilding is one of the most popular of all sports on the international level.

Through its member national federations, the IFBB oversees competitions in each nation, and it directly administers amateur and professional competition for men, women, and mixed pairs internationally.

INTENSITY

The degree of effort that you put into each set of your workout. The more intensity you place on a working muscle, the more quickly it will increase in hypertrophy. The most basic methods of increasing intensity are to use heavier weights in good form in each exercise, do more reps with a set weight, or perform a consistent number of sets and reps with a particular weight in a movement, but progressively reducing the length of rest intervals between sets.

ISOLATION EXERCISE

In contrast to a basic exercise, an isolation movement stresses a single muscle group (or sometimes just part of a single muscle) in relative isolation from the remainder of the body. Isolation exercises are good for shaping and defining various muscle groups. For your thighs: squats would be a typical basic movement. While leg extensions would be the equivalent isolation exercise.

JUICE

A slang term for anabolic steroids, e.g., being "on the juice."

LAYOFF

Most intelligent bodybuilders take a one or two-week layoff from bodybuilding training from time to time, during which they totally avoid the gym. A layoff after a period of intense pre-competition preparation is particularly beneficial as a means of allowing the body to completely rest, recuperate, and heal any minor training injuries that might have cropped up.

LIFTING BELT

This is a leather belt 3-5 inches wide at the back that is fastened tightly around your waist when you do squats, heavy back work, and overhead pressing movements. A lifting belt adds stability to your midsection, preventing lower back and abdominal injuries.

MASS

The size of the entire physique or the size of each muscle group. As long as you also have a high degree of muscularity and good balance of physical proportions, muscle mass is a highly prized quality among competitive bodybuilders.

MUSCULARITY

An alternative term for "definition" or "cuts."

NPC

The National Physique Committee Inc., which administers men's and women's amateur bodybuilding competitions in the United States. The NPC National Champions in each weight division are annually sent abroad to compete in the IFBB World Championships.

NUTRITION

The applied science of eating to foster greater health, fitness, and muscular grains. Through correct application of nutritional practices, you can selectively add muscle mass to your physique, or totally strip away all body fat, revealing the hard-earned muscles lying beneath your skin.

OLYMPIC BARBELL

A special type of barbell used in weightlifting and powerlifting competitions, but also used by bodybuilders in heavy basic exercises such as squats, bench presses, barbell be rows, standing barbell curls, standing barbell presses, and deadlifts. An Olympic barbell sans collars weighs 45 pounds, and each collar weighs five pounds.

OLYMPIC LIFTING

The type of weightlifting competition contested at the Olympic Games every four years, as well as at national and international competitions each year. Two lifts (the snatch and the clean jerk) are contested in a wide variety of weight classes.

OVERLOAD

The amount of weight that you force a muscle to use that is over and above its normal strength ability. Applying an overload to a muscle forces it to increase in hypertrophy.

PEAK

The absolute zenith of competitive condition achieved by a bodybuilder. To peak out optimally for a bodybuilding show, you must intelligently combine bodybuilding training, aerobic workouts, diet, mental conditioning, tanning, and a large number of other preparatory factors.

PLATES

The flat discs placed on the ends of barbell and dumbbell bars to increase the weight of the apparatus. Although some plates are made from vinyl-covered concrete, the best and most durable plates are manufactured from metal. Plates range in size from 1.25 - 100 pounds but using the term "plate" by itself refers to the 45 pounders.

POSE

Each individual stance that a bodybuilder does onstage in order to highlight his muscular development.

POUNDAGE

The amount of weight that you use in an exercise, whether that weight is on a barbell, dumbbell, or exercise machine.

POWER LIFTING

A second form of competitive weightlifting (not contested in the Olympics, however) featuring three lifts: The squat, bench press, and deadlift. Power lifting is contested both nationally and internationally in a wide variety of weight classes for both men and women.

PROGRESSION

The act of gradually adding to the amount of resistance that you use in each exercise. Without consistent progression in your workouts, you won't overload your muscles sufficiently to promote optimum increases in hypertrophy.

PUMP

The tight, blood-congested feeling in a muscle after it has been intensely trained. Muscle pump is caused by a rapid influx of blood into the muscles to remove fatigue toxins and replace supplies of fuel and oxygen. A good muscle pump is one of the indicators that show you have optimally worked a muscle group.

REPETITION (REP)

Each individual count of an exercise that is performed. Series of repetitions called "sets" are performed on each exercise in your training program.

RESISTANCE

The actual amount of weight that you are using in any exercise.

REST INTERVAL

The brief rest between sets that allows your body to partially recuperate prior to initiating the succeeding set. Usually between 1-5 minutes depending on how big the muscle group is.

RIPPED

The same as cut up.

ROUTINE

Also called a training schedule or program, a routine is the total list of exercise, sets, and reps (and sometimes weights) used in one training session.

SET

A grouping of repetitions that is followed by a rest interval and usually another set. Three to five sets are usually performed of each exercise.

SLEEVE

The hollow metal tube fit over the bar on most exercise barbell and dumbbell sets. This sleeve makes it easier for the bar to rotate in your hands as you do an exercise.

SPOTTERS

Training partners who stand by to act as safety helpers when you perform such heavy exercises as squats and bench presses. If you are stuck under and weight or begin to lose control of it, spotters can rescue you and prevent needless injuries.

STEROIDS

Prescription drugs which mimic male hormones, but without most of the androgenic side effects of actual testosterone. Many bodybuilders use these drugs to help increase muscle mass and strength.

STICKING POINT

A stalling out of bodybuilding progress. Also called a plateau.

STRETCHING

A type of exercise program in which you assume exaggerated postures that stretch muscles, joints, and connective tissues, hold these positions for several seconds, relax and then repeat the postures. Regular stretching exercise promotes body flexibility.

STRETCH MARKS

Tiny tears in a bodybuilder's skin caused by poor diet and in addition, rapid increases in bodyweight. If you notice stretch marks forming on your own body (usually around your pectoral-deltoid tie-ins), rub vitamin E cream over them two or three times per day, and try cutting back on your body weight by reducing body fat levels.

STRIATIONS

The tiny grooves of muscle across major muscle groups in a highly defined bodybuilder.

SUPERSETS

Series of two exercises performed with no rest between sets and a normal rest interval between supersets. Supersets increase training intensity by reducing the average length of rest interval between sets. They are also performed on the same muscle, not two different muscle groups.

SUPPLEMENTS

Concentrated vitamins, minerals, and proteins used by bodybuilders to improve the overall quality of their diets. Many bodybuilders believe that food supplements help to promote quality muscle growth.

SYMMETRY

The shape or general outline of a person's body, as when seen in silhouette. If you have good symmetry, you will have relatively wide shoulders, flaring lats, a small waist-hip structure, and generally small joints.

TESTOSTERONE

The male hormone primarily responsible for the maintenance of muscle mass and strength induced by heavy training. Testosterone is secondarily responsible for developing such secondary male sex characteristics as a deep voice, body hair, and male pattern baldness.

TRISETS

Series of three exercises performed with no rest between movements and a normal rest interval between trisets. Trisets increase training intensity by reducing the average length of rest interval between sets.

VASCULARITY

A prominence of veins and arteries over the muscles and beneath the skin of a sell-defined bodybuilder.

WARM-UP

The 5-15 minutes session of light calisthenics, aerobic exercise, and stretching taken prior to handling heavy bodybuilding training movements. A good warm-up helps to prevent injuries and actually allows you to get more out of your training than if you went into a workout cold.

WEIGHT

The same as Poundage or Resistance.

WEIGHTLIFTING

The competitive form of weight training in which each athlete attempts to lift as much as he can in well-defined exercises. Olympic lifting and power lifting are the two types of weightlifting competition.

WEIGHT TRAINING

An umbrella term used to categorize all acts of using resistance training. Weight training can be used to improve the body, rehabilitate injuries, improve sports conditioning, or as a competitive activity in terms of bodybuilding weightlifting.

WORKOUT

A bodybuilding or weight-training session.

###